My World is not Your World

Alison Hale

 Archimedes Press

First published in 1998 by Archimedes Press
Glebe House
Station Lane
Ingatestone
Essex CM4 0BP
United Kingdom

Reprinted 98

This book is sold subject to the condition that it shall not, by way of trade or otherwise, be lent, re-sold, hired out, or otherwise circulated without the publisher's prior consent in any form of binding or cover other than that in which it is published and without a similar condition including this condition being imposed on the subsequent purchaser.

Copyright © Alison Hale 1998

All rights reserved. No part of this document may be reprinted or reproduced, or utilised in any form by electronic, mechanical or other means, now known or hereafter invented, including photocopying and recording, or in any information storage and retrieval system, without permission in writing from Archimedes Press.

For all the children and adults suffering from and working with those who suffer from similar problems.

Acknowledgements

Thank you to my parents and sister for their perseverance and support throughout my life and during the writing of my book. Thank you to Valerie for her encouragement, meticulously correcting my grammar and for being a good sounding-board during the months when I was engrossed in finding the words to express my world. My thanks to Edna, Sheila C. and Sheila M. for their constructive criticism and words of encouragement and also to Irene and Jenny C. during the final stages of the creation of this book. Lastly, thank you to all those who have supported and spurred me on during my life.

...and many thanks to my computer, for without your help this would have never been written...

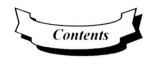

Preface	6
1. Turmoil	8
2. Living on the edge	14
3. Separations	48
4. Marooned in desolation	63
5. Finding a way	72
6. Confrontation	91
7. Building bridges	99
8. Moving out into the world	119

Preface

Why does the Universe exist?
Why do humans exist?
Do humans have the intellectual capacity to understand the Universe?
If there is a point to human life, what is it?
I often ponder such questions although I do not expect to answer them within my lifetime; but I do believe that everyone should make the most of everything they have within their own situation, without exploitation. This philosophy of life is the underlying driving force behind this book. I wish to share my 26 years of firsthand experience of living in a world where all I perceive is distorted, so that others, like myself, can have the opportunity for a much better deal out of life. Since with knowledge comes understanding and with understanding comes tolerance and then the chance to flourish.

Since my teenage years it has been generally recognised by the professionals that I suffer from Dyslexia. However, as I describe my world in this book, connections with other related disorders such as Dyspraxia, Attention Deficit Disorder, Autism seem to emerge. It also shows the potential for secondary neurosis such as Agoraphobia. (I give a more detailed account of all these conditions in part 8.) As in all science that is moving forward, in answering a few questions, many more will be raised which as yet are unanswered. I am not a definitive authority on these disabilities, merely a sufferer from aspects of them. However, the insight this book gives can be used to gain a more informed approach to understanding others like myself.

Many with this disability perceive in similar or parallel ways and use strategies to help overcome some of the problems. My strategies/compensations may not be the same as those of someone else but there will be analogous elements. This insight has made me take a second look at others with similar problems and has made me try and understand how they perceive, feel and compensate. For many people, one of the most confusing aspects, is that a person may suffer from one or many of the individual parts which make up any of the fore-mentioned conditions. In other words, there are a huge number of different combinations that can occur and these happen in varying degrees. For instance, a person may suffer from Dyslexia but may also have Dyspraxic tendencies. Alternatively, another may suffer from some or all problems in each area. Such diversity of symptoms makes accurate diagnosis very hard. There are a great many potential pitfalls for the unenlightened.

There are numerous experienced researchers, doctors, psychologists, educationalists, teachers and parents who have spent many years dealing with people in general and with people such as myself. Many of these professionals believe that they know what we are experiencing, but their research, observations and learning all come from second hand experience. These professionals, who do not suffer from these problems, are at a distinct disadvantage and regretfully very often make a whole string of false assumptions, based on their second or third hand experience, resulting in them misinterpreting and consequently misunderstanding the problems. Often these professional people find it hard to accept new ways of looking at and thinking about these problems. I would like these professionals to listen to those of us who can say exactly what we perceive from our own first hand experience.

Although I am severely dyslexic, this book has been written by myself, but has been grammatically corrected by outsiders. My English is not the most eloquent, but expressing all that has happened in my own words ensures that no one distorts my experiences. Born in 1969 into a middle class family, I grew up in a medium sized village in the south east of England. I lived with both my natural parents and sister throughout this time. The book follows from childhood my struggles in trying to bridge the gap between 'my world', and 'the world' in which I was expected to live, with its constraints and expectations.

The book is comprised of many of my most dominant memories, to help build up a picture of my way of comprehending 'the world'. I attended mainstream state schools throughout my school life and have never received any additional help before, during or after leaving school in any form, other than some ordinary (not specifically for Dyslexia sufferers) remedial English lessons. Throughout the whole of my childhood and most of my teens, apart from my Dyslexia, nobody realised there was anything else medically wrong with me. I was simply perceived as odd, different. One important point to note is that until very recently I have not had enough language ability to express exactly how I am. On the whole I thought everybody perceived the same way as I do and everyone else thought that my perceptions were like theirs. These were incorrect and misleading assumptions. I had no frame of reference other than myself and therefore could not verbalise my unusual perceptions. As a consequence I normally appeared slow and stupid. It was not until reaching the age of 17 that I and my immediate family began to explore and realise that the way I perceive 'the world' is actually quite different from that of most people. As the years progressed I slowly gained good frames of reference and was able to unravel and then express the mysteries of my world.

This book is written from my perspective and shows how distorted my perception of the world was. Unfortunately many of the people mentioned frequently come across in a very unfavourable light. My book is not in any way a criticism of any person mentioned. The people featured in my book are not in any way bad, incompetent or insensitive, they are just ordinary people who did not have the knowledge to understand my situation, which in turn caused us all to misinterpret, misunderstand and misconceive each other. Given the same circumstances, I do not believe that anyone could have done any better without fully understanding my perspective of 'the world'.

..please, come into 'my world' and just for a moment completely forget your world...

ONE

Turmoil

1

....aged three to five....in the beginning all was not calm....

I feel terror struck. It is one of those mornings yet again. They seem to come around so often, too often; it does not matter how scared I feel and how much I cry, they always take me there. I am being transported to that place, the vast place where the screams, voices, the bangs, the footsteps combine to make this painfully deafening confusing mush of sound. Although as we walk in the tears run down my face, nobody seems to notice my terror as the noise consumes me and the multicoloured blurs rush past me screaming, shouting and sometimes knocking me. The only reassuring safe reference point in all this chaos is fast moving towards the door. Why does my mother insist on leaving me here? Once she has gone I will be isolated in this confusion for what will seem like an eternity. Although one or two of my friends are here in this bedlam, it is very hard to distinguish anything, let alone find one of them in amongst all these moving blurs. If I can be with one of them this gives me a minute sense of security, which is better than nothing. My friends and family call this place Play School, I think of it more in terms of 'Terror' School.

    After a while I normally manage to compose myself in the knowledge that I will eventually be allowed out of this prison. The doors are locked so that we cannot escape and the bottoms of the windows are way above my head. Today it is my turn to do the painting. We are given this large sheet of glaring white paper on which to paint. I know that to remove this painful glare all I have to do is to paint the whole sheet of paper black. For some reason nobody, including my mother, ever seems enamoured with my completely black paintings. Strangely, they try to make me use a confusion of dazzling bright colours.

    Normally towards the end of the morning we all have to sit down quietly and have a drink. At last these blurs of colour stay in one place and the volume of sound subsides to a mumbling. In the comparative stillness and reduced noise I begin to feel a sense of calm coming over me. Finally we sit in a circle. We must be quiet and only one person speaks, a lady who, I think, tells a story, but it is hard for me to understand the strange sounds in this voice, which is foreign to me. It works both ways, because the grown-ups do not understand me when I speak. I know that soon for one more awful moment the blurs will start rushing around again causing that terrible confusion, but at least at this point my mother will be coming to take me back to the comparable safety of our home. Relative peace at last.

It is bad enough going to 'Terror' School with my mother but this morning I am being taken there by a friend's mother. A wave of dread engulfs me and the tears are dripping down my face as we drive off round the corner. The car stops abruptly outside another friend's house. Apparently we are also giving him a lift to Play School. Suddenly and without warning he runs, straight through the glass of the closed front door! (He was not seriously injured) Wow, what a wonderful way of avoiding going to 'Terror' School and making all the grown-ups rush around madly! If he does not have to go, why should I? Hopefully, now we will not have to go. My hope is short lived, the disappointment is overwhelming and my tears once again flood down my face as we arrive at the door of the 'Terror' School. Despite the fact that some of the other children are offering me their toys to play with, all I want to do is go home. I am in luck, as my friend's mother is going to take me home.

As we arrive home I am so thankful and just cry through sheer relief that I did not have to stay in the bedlam. Surely, my mother will now realise how awful it is at 'Terror' School and therefore I will never have to go there again. It does not matter how much I protest, my mother is adamant that I should continue going to Play School. Why does she make me go to such a horrible place? My mother tells me that my friend ran through the front door because he was so excited and could not wait to go to Play School. She must mistaken. My mother also tells me that my friends enjoy going to Play School and therefore I should also like it. I cannot understand how this can be true but, if this is it and my friends do actually enjoy their time at 'Terror' School, they must be very peculiar.

After what has felt like an eternity, the wonderful day has come when we are at the 'Terror' School for the final time. I am absolutely delighted that I will never have to return to this horribly confusing and disorientating place, with the crushing noise and manic multicoloured blurs. Strangely, for some reason, which completely escapes me, many of my peers are crying their little eyes out. I cry because I hate coming here but they are crying because we will never have to come here again! It does not make any sense. At last I am free of the anarchy and burden of 'Terror' School. Could Primary School be as bad as Play School? It could not be, could it? No, surely not.

2

....thrust forward into an education system which appears only to cope with the 'average normal' pupil.... At this point in time, people only existed when they were with me. I went as a rising 5-year-old to primary school and would therefore have to do 3 years of infant classes. I spent 2 years at my first Primary school.

I am told this is the day that most people never forget. I dearly hope that going to Primary school will be less traumatic then 'Terror' school. We are filed into a classroom, each with our respective mother. This is much better than that large Hall of the 'Terror' School and all the multicoloured blurs are relatively quiet and still. This really is not too bad. We are asked by the teacher to sit round on the carpeted floor in the corner of the room. Where is my mother? She's gone! Leaping to my feet I run towards the door as fast as my little legs will take me,

"Come back", shouts the teacher as she runs towards the door. I grab the door handle and feel her hand come crashing down on top of mine.

"Mummy can't have gone far, I can catch her up!" I exclaim. The teacher says my mother has gone home and she will not let me go and find her. I hate the teacher for tricking my mother and me. If I had known that my mother was leaving I would have gone with her. Now I am alone in this strange place, disorientated, lost, frightened and crying. My mother, who was my only reliable reference point, has gone. Despite making every excuse I can think up the teacher refuses to let me go home. As the day has worn on things have worsened. The multicoloured blurs have started rushing around, chattering, shouting, and screaming. The noise is deafening and I cannot cope with this chaotic environment. When will we be allowed to leave this dreadful place and go home?

After that terrible first day, every day seemed to run into the next. It was just one long round of me trying each morning not to go to school, crying all the way to school and during the first part of the day. Each day we were squashed into a chair behind a table. Each day the multicoloured blurs raced around making a crushing noise. Each day I had trouble finding my friends, children who I could rely on as a reference point. Each day I was disorientated and confused. Each day at an unpredictable time, we were all bundled into the turmoil of the deafening dining hall and crowded round the tables. For the first few days of my school life I was permitted by the teacher to stay in the classroom while the others went outside to the playground. But from then on she insisted that each day, we were all periodically thrust outside into the vast bewildering blur of blinding grey and green areas, where all the multicoloured blurs dashed around. Finally, each day we would be allowed home, but I carried the appalling knowledge that I would have to return to this bedlam. My mother's insistence that I should go to school is completely unreasonable and cruel. I cannot understand why she or anybody else should think that school is a 'nice' place; they must all be very stupid.

After a few months I started to learn to suppress my emotional response to the continuing frightening situation at school and also managed to make some stable references, for example one or two friends, my desk and a particular area of the playground. These things gave me a tiny sense of security in my chaotic environment. I am always falling over, too often says the dinner lady. The only good aspect about falling over and grazing my knees is that I have to go inside to the school nurse. It is quiet and peaceful in her office. Many times I took the drastic measure of cutting my knees with my fingernails or some stones just so that I could go into the peace and quiet.

I mostly ignore the teachers. They do not hold my respect and hardly ever say anything worth listening to. The words are not tangible, so have little meaning and therefore are of no use to me. That is, when I can hear what they are saying. Usually they just make a garbled rubbishy mush of blurry noises; how do they expect us to understand such weird language? Still, at least things are equal, because sometimes the teacher (and other grown-ups) cannot work out what I am saying. I wish that teachers would not torture the whole class for being corporately noisy. We are made to put our hands on our heads. Do we really deserve excruciating pain in our arms, shoulders, necks and backs?

Periodically we are sent to different rooms e.g. the Hall, classroom next door. I do not understand why a person's voice changes relative to a room (with different acoustics). In each different room the same teacher's voice completely changes and often becomes totally incomprehensible. When we go to the room next door we are always asked to take some things with us, e.g. a pencil, but I never seem to understand the teachers garbled instructions and always without fail, arrive without the appropriate writing implements. The teacher often crossly says,

"You would forget your own head if it wasn't screwed on". I do not understand how a person's head is 'screwed' on! Or indeed how to 'screw' a person's head off. Once in the other classroom the other teacher comes in and often plays the piano, but she is always talking about the 'high' and 'low' sounds/notes. She often plays a note and then asks,

"Was that a high or a low sound/note?"

Over many weeks I have very closely examined the piano at home and the one at school and still I cannot see which end of the piano keyboard is the furthest from the floor. After all it is logical that a 'high' note should be 'higher' up off the floor and conversely a 'low' note should be 'closer' to the floor, therefore the keyboard should be tilted. I have even sat looking straight at the piano to remove any foreshortening effects, but the keyboard still appears to lie completely parallel to the floor. I really cannot see which side of the keyboard is furthest from the floor. Since I am unable to see which end of the piano is at the highest altitude how can I possibly see whether she is playing a 'high' or 'low' note? Maybe, if I keep on looking, one day I will be able to see which is the higher end of the keyboard on the piano?

I have noticed that many of my peers are reading, but to me reading is a total mystery. Should I be looking at the black bits that disappear and then reappear or the white bits that also disappear and then reappear? Which is the most prominent, is it the black or the white? Is it the shapes of the black areas I should read, or should I look at the spaces between the black i.e. read the white? It is just completely baffling. The white bits form moving rivers that flow in between the black bits. Then to be even more confusing the teacher uses a blackboard, but we write on and read from, white paper. So what should I read when looking at the blackboard, is it different? When we write we inscribe the black onto the white. Is this so we can read the black letters? Or do we inscribe the black onto the white so that it makes gaps in the white, so allowing us to read the white? How have my friends discovered whether to read the black or the white? I have asked my teachers, parents and friends,

"What should I read?" But I never manage to find a satisfactory answer. They never seem to understand my enquiry. (At this time I could not manipulate the English language adequately to express my confusion). Besides, who needs to read anyway? It is obvious to me that I am the cleverest person in the class, despite not being able to read!

I can without any trouble outwit any of my peers and the teacher. When we play 'hide and seek' in the playground, I of course keep my eyes open when I am supposed to be the one doing the seeking and counting. Obviously if I shut my eyes I will fall over or if I am leaning against something I will become dizzy. So I pretend to shut my eyes just leaving a little slit for me to see through, which means I am able to see at the very least in which direction my friends are going to be hiding in. I do not understand how or why most of my friends actually shut their eyes! It seems very odd, but if they wish to do something so daft who am I to stop them! When I am the one doing the hiding I often initially run in the opposite direction and then double back on myself so that the one doing the counting does not know where I am going. Why my friends have not thought of this I really do not know!

Often I play my games with the teacher, for example only the other day I acquired a large lump of 'blu tac'. It is wonderful stuff, it feels different under different conditions and is very versatile. The teacher confiscated my large piece of 'blu tac' and took it to her desk, but very foolishly left it on her desk while she listened to one pupil at a time reading. I have decided that when it is my turn to go and read I will open my book and put it down reasonably hard on top of the 'blu tac', using the side of the book furthest away from her. I know that her desk is relatively rough and that my book has a shiny back and therefore the 'blu tac' will stick to my book rather than the desk. Whilst reading I will have to hold the book carefully, since it will not be possible to rest it flat on the desk with a large lump of 'blu tac' on the back cover! When I have finished reading to the teacher I will carefully slide the book off the table at such an angle that she will not see the 'blu tac'. I executed this without any trouble. Unfortunately, later in the afternoon someone saw me with the 'blu tac' and that goody-two-shoes told the teacher! The teacher promptly came over to me and confiscated the 'blu tac' and I was very pleased with myself, because she told me she had no idea how I managed to remove the 'blu tac' from her desk! I do not care that she now has the 'blu tac' because it has been worth it to confirm to myself that I am much more intelligent than the teacher is.

When we are in the playground near the teachers stationary parked cars, we stop and look at the cars because they are moving! If I for once in my life, stand still and look at these cars they seem to be moving back and forth, up and down and from side to side. How can this be? Objects do not move unless something moves them; so what force is moving these cars? Now that I come to think of it many objects move around in an inexplicable way when I stop and look at them. Maybe, I have a special power and can move objects with my mind? The problem is, I cannot seem to control where they move to and they never seem to move very far from their original position. After I have tried to move an object and have seen it moving, it always seems to be back where it started; or has it moved a smidgen? Perhaps, as I grow up I will be able to move the objects properly with my mind?

I look forward to 'going home time' at the end of the day. As we walk from the school towards the waiting parents, a sea of faces confronts us, most of the mothers look about the same. Distinguishing my mother is a very difficult task. Still, if I cannot find her she comes and grabs me. Free at last, free to do what I want, free to be me. I can do what I like, within reason. Play with the objects called friends outside our house, play with the irritating little sister, build or create something or just watch a television programme. When we play I am in charge and decide what we are going to do and how. This is my time of learning when I can discover how things work, how things look and how things feel, particularly how hard things are. I pick things up, play with them, feel them, squash them, hit them or take them apart. Anything tangible will do as long as I can interact with it and learn about it. In addition, I am able to experiment with manipulating these objects called people and see if I can make them do what I wish. I do not care what any object is called. It is irrelevant. The only aspect, which is relevant, is what it does and therefore I never remember the names of any of the objects including these called children. There is no point.

Any adult whom I find to be a reasonable person gives me the same amount of security as my mother. The amount of security a person can offer me is the only important thing about them. My mother says that I must change schools, hopefully the teachers will be stupid so that I can carry on doing what I like at school. Perhaps the new school will be less chaotic?

After spending two years at school I had learnt very little and was performing well below average in most disciplines including basic reading, writing and mathematics. There were of course the usual hassles at home, disagreements with my parents, some deliberately naughty behaviour on my part and fights with my sister, but nothing beyond the 'norm'.

TWO

Living On The Edge

I

.....*September 1976. Final year in an infant class. I was aged 7 for most of this academic year... Having spent my first 2 years at school without learning anything academic, my parents started to become worried. The schoolteachers did not seem to be overly concerned. Perhaps I was a 'slow starter' and would catch up later? Maybe my intelligence was lower than my parents wanted to believe? They decided that I should change schools and spend the final year of my infant school life and the whole of my junior school life in a smaller Primary school in an adjacent village. When we visited the school, my parents found the headmistress to be the sort of person who liked and was really interested in children. My parents felt that the slightly smaller class sizes would give me a better chance of making progress and the education system an opportunity to give me the help and encouragement I apparently needed. The school had two infant classes and 4 junior classes. I spent the first year in the top infant class then spent one year in each of the junior classes.*

My mother yelled out,

"Come on Alison, hurry up. We don't want to be late. Now you are not going to cry, are you? There is absolutely no reason to cry. You are a big girl now. Don't you dare cry. Remember you are a big girl now!". Her voice cuts through me like ice, why does she not realise how petrified I feel? Yes, of course she must; I suppose? My tears are the only medium I have for expressing my fear. I expect this new school will be as manically chaotic as the previous one and that really scares me. I can still remember the fear I felt during my first days at the other Primary school. This time my terror is consuming me as we drive down the road to the school and we have not even arrived there yet. I must concentrate on controlling my emotional response to this fear. I MUST NOT CRY, I Must Not Cry, I will not cry.........

The clutter and confusion in the classroom overwhelm me. My desk is my space and reference point but it is situated in the middle of complete disorder. My whole mind is consumed with trying to control my terror and trying to control my emotional response to that terror. The day seems to be never ending, but finally we have been allowed out and I am reunited with my mother. I have not cried all day and am very proud of my achievement and said to my mother with joy and relief,

"Mummy I did not cry all day!"

"I should think not", she mumbled and continued on with what she was doing. I have spent the whole day making sure that I did not cry so that she would not be disappointed with me. Why is she not pleased with me? Why is she not proud of me? What more could I have done?

As time has progressed I have made some stable references: one or two friends, my desk, coat hook, a corner of the playground. These references take the sharp edge off the all-consuming bedlam. My infant school teacher does not seem to me to be too stupid or too clever, she appears to be a reasonable sort of person. I can tolerate her. I just wish that when she wrote on the blackboard, she did not make such a mess. She cannot even write in a straight line, the lines of writing wiggle across the blackboard at varying tilts. We are expected to accurately copy these letters from the words! It would be much easier to copy if I knew which letters belonged to which word and which words belonged to which line. Despite trying very hard I am often in trouble for being careless when I copy from the blackboard, but surely it is the teacher who should get told off for messiness.

Unfortunately it is Monday morning yet again. Each Monday it is the same, we are told to write a few sentences about our weekend. The problem is, as usual I have no frame of reference and therefore have no idea what I was doing yesterday, let alone the day before. What I did at the weekend is completely irrelevant! The here and now is the only thing which is relevant. I guess I will have to make up something, which I might have feasibly been doing last weekend. I have purposely broken my pencil lead several times and spent much time re-sharpening the pencil and even more time chatting to anyone who will listen. I have now decided to scribe a few letters onto the page. I always try my best to write something sensible, neatly and spelt to the best of my ability.

The teacher said softly and calmly,

"What is this. I can't read this. You have not left any gaps between the words!" Whoops! I have forgotten about the gaps again. The teacher does not appear too worried and said,

"Tell me what you have written".

"I don't know". Oh dear, as usual I cannot remember what I have written because it was completely immaterial and trivial. It's not fair. The teacher has told me to restart this piece of work and to leave gaps between the words. This is so infuriating. Why should my work be redone? I have tried my best! Often in books and on the blackboard it is hard to see where the gaps are and sometimes the gaps are non-existent so why should I use gaps? It is so ridiculous! Even when I do leave gaps, often the teacher cannot read the way I spell words. Spelling is a complete mystery to me. Why is there a convention for spelling? Why can we not spell words any way we like?

Periodically we must all go and read to the teacher. For the first time I have been given a choice over which type of book to read, and have chosen a book about pirates. The fascinating pictures are the best part. The words in the book defeat me. I am still unsure whether to read the black patterns or the white patterns. I do not understand why 'island' is not pronounced 'is' - 'land'? This is one of the very few words that I can actually read. Last week my father told me off for being unable to read the word 'are', he said if you say the middle letter, that is the way the word is pronounced. If this is so why not just write the letter, r? Why bother with the other two letters? The English language seems to lack any consistency; it seems to have a completely random construction.

This afternoon, I will, via some devious actions, try to determine who is the cleverest; me or the teacher. At the end of the afternoon it is story-time and we must sit still and quietly whilst the teacher reads. Quite frankly it is a relief that all the multicoloured blurs are quiet and still. At least when it is this quiet it is possible to hear some of the words and parts of words which are being read, enough for me to deduce something about the story. The story is vaguely interesting in parts but this bit is boring me to death. My plan is to pretend to do some writing. I believe that the teacher should know by now how much I detest writing and therefore she should be able to deduce that I am messing around and purposely trying to trick her! I move my head very near to the desk, bring one arm around so that it is covering most of the pretend piece of paper and start moving my other hand around as if I were writing very small with an extremely short pencil.

Ha, ha, the teacher has fallen into my trap! I do not care that she is shouting at me. Oh, what a shame! She seems to be cross! Well I will not shatter this good illusion. Opening the desk lid very carefully I pretend to slide the small piece of paper into the desk and then simulate placing a pencil in the desk, stand up and proudly walk out of the classroom. I believe the teacher should have known that I would never voluntarily do writing, therefore I conclude that she is not as clever as I am. Anyway, I like being sent out of the classroom because I can sit in the lovely stillness of the corridor. It is peaceful out here and if I so desire I can still hear enough words of the story to understand the general gist. Alternatively, I can sit and contemplate the universe.

I have this wonderful and beautiful little magazine cutting of a spiral galaxy. I find it completely fascinating and the idea of all the stars making this galaxy which is so far away is riveting. I want to understand this fascinating, beautiful Universe; so big, so many stars and we can see some of the stars at night. I want to be a part of the spiral galaxy. I try to conceptualise how the universe works and how a God may fit into it, but my thoughts are far beyond my verbal skills. It would be great if I could discuss these thoughts with an adult. Someone said God is everywhere on Earth and has something to do with hearts - I wish I knew the words to ask whether God is intermingled with the air we breath and therefore gets into our hearts? If God were part of the air this would also explain how God is everywhere simultaneously.

Obviously everyone's face looks virtually the same and the way of distinguishing one person from another is by his or her hairstyle. What is going on? That is not my mother! My mother's hair is shoulder length and is straight except at the bottom where it curls up and out. Her hair is not this short and curled under at the bottom. There is an intruder in our house. It cannot possibly be my mother, as her hair is longer and somehow different.

"Hallo June", said Shirley Nana[1]. Has Shirley Nana not noticed that this is a different person, does she not even recognise that this is not her own daughter? Does she realise that her daughter does not have her hair like that? This is all very confusing. Surely my father will notice the difference when he comes home from work.

"Hallo", said my father as he came in and planted a kiss on the cheek of the lady masquerading as my mother. It is true that the intruder does look very similar to my mother but the hairstyle is wrong. My father must know about the deception, he must have trained this lady to act like my mother so that the rest of us would not notice. It seems to have worked as far as my sister Jenny and Shirley Nana are concerned. They do not appear to have noticed the change in hairstyle. It does not fool me, I know that cannot possibly be my mother. This is terrifying. I think it would be unwise to let my father know that I realise what is going on, because he may replace me in the same way that my mother has been replaced! What has happened to my real mother? When is this intruder going to slip up and accidentally reveal her true identity? Hopefully my real mother can come back soon. I hope they do not expect me to like this intruder?

Nobody, not even Aunty, seemed to notice that mum had been replaced.

"Lets teach Jenny some nursery rhymes", said Aunty. Well I know for a fact that Jenny knows most of them already. The problem is I do not know any nursery rhymes, they mean nothing to me, and they are complete nonsense. Why would anyone want to learn such meaningless sets of words? However, Aunty is unaware that I do not know any nursery rhymes and neither do I want her to know. If only I could find the words to describe the irrelevance of nursery rhymes and explain to Aunty that their repetition is pointless and therefore they must be intended for idiots. So there is only one logical reply to her request about teaching Jenny some nursery rhymes and that is,

"No, nursery rhymes are silly".

"Come on Alison, don't be like that", replied Aunty. After she and Shirley Nana started singing the rhymes, Jenny quickly joined them.

"Alison, don't be so silly", said Aunty, "do them with us". Even if I want to say those silly words, I cannot remember the order. Why would I want to repeat such nonsense? Now Shirley Nana is obviously irritated and has announced that I am sulking and has told the others to ignore me. It is best that they think that I am being awkward, at least while they are ignoring me they will leave me alone. They might mock me if they realise that the words of rhymes elude me. Why do they place such importance on irrelevant things?

I cannot read, write, add up (addition) or take away (subtraction). It does not bother me, for I have no reason to be able to do anything that involves English or

---

[1] As a child this was the name I gave to my maternal grandmother and will continue to use it throughout this book.

Maths because they seem to have no practical use. Unfortunately, my father disagrees. Why, I really cannot imagine? To me this whole counting game is worthless. Why would anyone need to be able to count to 100?

"You aren't going out to play until you have learnt to count to one hundred" said my father very firmly. This is ridiculous, we do these irrelevant number games at school, why do we also have to do them at home?

"Right", said my father, "how far can you get". So I start,

"1, 2, 3,..., 19, er, 20, 21, 22,..., 29, er, 30, 31,..., 39, er, 60"

"NO not 60, 40 comes next", said my father. I continue on,

"40, 41,..., 49, er, 60?"

"NO, No not 60, 50 comes next" said my father. I carry on,

"50, 51,..., 59, er, 60?"

"Yes, hurry up, of course it's 60", he is starting to become cross. I proceed,

"60, 61,..., 69, er, 80?"

"NO, NO it's 70" he growled. I am going to be in big trouble in a minute if I am not careful.

"70, 71,..., 79, er, 100?", I exclaimed.

"For goodness sake 80 comes next", he said, becoming even more impatient. I had forgotten about 80.

"80, 81,..., 89, 100", I said proudly reaching the end at last.

"What about 90?" he shouted as he started to go red in the face.

"90, 91,..., 99, 100" surely this must now be the end, now I can go out to play.

"..and... where do you think you are going? Come back here. You are NOT going out to play until you have learnt to count to 100 properly", yelled my father. Composing himself, he said,

"This is the order 10, 20, 30, 40, 50, 60, 70, 80, 90, 100", now you say it. It is all very well him asking me to repeat after him, but I cannot remember what he has just said. I have no frame of reference by which to retain the order. We continued going round and round in ever decreasing circles for ages with my father becoming increasingly angry with me. Although I have tried with all my might to memorize the order, it was hopeless, for I have no way of remembering something without a tangible reference.

"Go on, you can go out to play now", he said to me despairingly. Standing up, I rush outside before he changes his mind! Now I am free to go and investigate the world around me and find out what sense I can make of all the millions of sensations, which surround and bombard me, then see how I can manipulate them! Perhaps I can play with some of those objects called children and find out what I can make them do! I hope there are no dogs outside. Dogs are really horrible, because they rush around haphazardly and make random intermittent loud noises. There is no way of knowing what they might do next.

At last I have come to the end of my first academic year at this loathsome school. In September I will be entering my first year as a junior. A goody-two-shoes 'friend' who has had the first year junior teacher for the last year has told me that the teacher is an 'ogre'! Hopefully this is an exaggeration. We will also have a new Headmistress. Will she be as friendly as the out going Headmistress and give us lots of sweets?

2

....*First Year Junior School.* I was aged 8 for most of this academic year.... I entered this class still unable to read more than a very few words. On a good day I could count to 100 and obtain the correct answers to very simple addition and subtraction sums. We had been introduced to simple multiplication tables but they appeared to be a set of numbers with no apparent connection, consequently I was unable to master them. At this time my parents were becoming increasingly concerned with my lack of progress. They wondered if I was of low intelligence or just a slow starter. But, having seen and heard comments about this condition called Dyslexia, they began, unbeknown to me, to wonder if this was my problem. At this time, Dyslexia was considered by the many involved in the education system (including many teachers), to be a figment of the imagination of middle class parents whose expectations exceeded the ability of their intellectually incapable children. The parents of such children believed their children had at least good average intelligence since they were able to do many things, but had specific trouble learning to read, write, remember, tell the time, learn left from right etc. Unfortunately, this real and physical problem of Dyslexia was often patronisingly branded by many as a 'middle class disorder'. As far as I am aware, throughout my school life, I never received any specific educational help designed to assist people with Dyslexia. I was being 'taught' to read and spell using the 'look and say' method. Could the right sort of help early on have enabled me to excel?

Nerves are beginning to engulf me. That nasty day has come, the day I return to school to start the new school year. I hate school because it is just one long struggle in chaos. To make it worse my little sister Jenny is going to school for her first day. I can barely read. My worst fear is that Jenny may be like my friends and be good at reading. If she is good at reading she will show me up. I wish I could read it would make my life much easier.

"Now Alison, take care of Jenny today won't you?" said my mother in a concerned voice. Nobody took care of me on my first day at either school and in fact my mother did not even care that I had not cried on my first day at this school. Why therefore should she want me to molly-coddle Jenny? There is only one logical reply to my mother's ridiculous request,

"NO WAY. Anyway, the infants use a different playground to the juniors, thank goodness!"

In this new classroom I have my own desk and therefore can start building some stable references. Like many places this classroom is very painfully noisy. All the piercingly loud sounds bombard me. There are so many children in this classroom that we have been jammed in tightly. This teacher seems to keep shouting. I hate shouting; it hurts my ears and interrupts my thoughts. Anyone who slightly misbehaves seems to be in big trouble. This is a problem. I have just had a brilliant idea. At the moment, the only way I am going to be able to manipulate this teacher so that I can do what I like, without getting into trouble, is by observing her every move really carefully. Find out exactly what others in my class can get away with and observe who gets into trouble and why; plus discover exactly what her punishments are. This way I will know exactly where her weak points and boundaries lie and this analysis will enable me to further investigate my environment my way, whilst avoiding getting into trouble.

Nothing this teacher says seems to me to make any sense. For instance, the teacher spoke about 'floors'; I cannot imagine how people have 'floors' inside them or how 'floors' make people imperfect or what 'floors' have to do with some people having one ear lower than the other! It all seems very weird.[2]

For many weeks we have been working through these silly confusing textbooks, they rarely make any sense to me. The words are impossible to read. Today the teacher has asked us to do a particular exercise. There is a strip of four cartoon pictures and some captions. The object is to put the appropriate caption under each picture. This seems to me to be a daft request by the teacher. I cannot read the words or see what is depicted on each of these line drawing cartoon pictures. Having studied both the pictures and the captions for a while, I am no closer to finding which belongs to which. There must be a reasonable chance that if I guess, I should get at least one of them in the correct place, so that is what I have done. I have often guessed in the past, with varying amounts of success.

A few days later, the teacher told the whole class that most of them had done the exercise well. Unfortunately for me, she revealed to the whole class that I had made a disgraceful mess and that if I had taken more notice and care over my work, this would not have happened. I have been told to redo this exercise. I hate this teacher and dislike any teacher who reprimands me in front of the whole class. I dare not tell the teacher, but I know that I tried very hard, how dare she imply that I am careless and stupid. Staring at the exercise again does not seem to help, for neither the cartoon pictures or the words make any sense. Nobody sitting near me will tell me the correct answers.

As usual, I am in trouble for chatting. Little does the teacher know that I am trying to bargain with anyone who has the correct answers to this silly exercise. I seem unable to persuade anyone to give me the answers so there is no option but to guess again, especially since the teacher is starting to ask why I have not yet

---

[2] The teacher was referring to 'flaws'.

finished the exercise. I know that it is improbable that I will guess them all right, but at least I have increased my chances by knowing that what I did last time was wrong. Just to get one right will be better than nothing.

Finally I made my guesses and found enough courage to take them to the teacher. I am sure the whole class must have heard her express her disbelief at all my answers still being incorrect. She seems to think that I have not paid any attention and have been purposely careless. Why does this teacher never seem to understand me? Why does the teacher never seem to help me? Why does she seem to treat me as if I am completely brainless? What should I do? There is no way that I can work out which picture belongs to which caption. I need to convince someone with the correct answers to give them to me. It is incredibly difficult to persuade anyone to divulge the answers because they fear getting into trouble with the teacher. After much pleading I did manage to persuade someone to give me the answers.

The teacher does not realise how I obtained the answers and is pleased that I have finally done the exercise properly!! She seems to think that when I concentrate I can do my work properly! Even though I now have the correct answers they mean nothing. I still have no idea what the words say or what the pictures show. This teacher appears to have no tolerance or respect for me as a person and I feel nothing but contempt towards her.

I detest reading to the teacher, every time it seems to be the same scenario. We are all in 'reading groups' each with about 5 children and I am at the bottom of the lowest group, which makes me the worst person in the whole class. In amongst all the deafening noise and moving chaos of the classroom we all have to stand around in a semicircle facing the teacher and are expected to concentrate and listen to each other reading! Which is daft because I have not learnt to hear individual voices in a noisy environment, where a voice is just part of the mixture of sounds. Each page contains several sentences and we each must take our turn at reading a page.

I cannot hear what the others are saying, or read any of the words in the book and therefore when it is my turn I never know when or where to start. Despite trying my hardest, the teacher becomes annoyed and despairs at my apparent lack of concentration, which in turn gives me a sense of uselessness. I know that I read extremely slowly and in fact I even have great difficulty recognising the very few words which I can read. At least today I know what the first word is, so I start reading,

"No, ...umm". Yet again I seem to have made the teacher angry, apparently I should have known that the word was 'on'. I do not mean to irritate the teacher. We continue to go through every word in this way. First I try and read the word, then the teacher tells me what the word actually says. Finally after what seems like an eternity of torture we reach the end of the few sentences which I have to read. The teacher normally tells me to go back to the beginning of my few sentences and reread them to the group and today is no exception. So I cast my eyes back to the beginning. I cannot remember any of the words. Every time I look at them they look different because the white and black patterns are forever changing. How does anyone ever remember the infinite number of patterns per word? We go through the whole ugly scene again with me trying to read each word, then the teacher telling me what the word actually says. I find it so frustrating and humiliating and the teacher often remarks that I should have concentrated the first time through the passage. Even after going through the passage a second time I have no idea what these fragmented sentences are about, so how am I supposed to remember the words?

Even when I am asked to read the passage for a third time I am still unable to read it much better than on my first attempt. My lack of ability seems to make the teacher furious. Often she comments that my silliness affects the whole 'reading group' and prevents them from progressing with their reading. It is a great relief when the teacher asks the next person to start reading because at least while they are reading her attention is deflected from me.

So I cannot read. Is it really the end of the world? When I am grown up I will become an artist, because artists paint pictures and therefore do not need to read. The Headmistress, who is also our art teacher, says my paintings are very good. I like painting. These days there is a specific purpose to painting. We are often told to paint a picture of a tangible object or scene. Since the purpose of painting is to paint an object, I no longer simply paint the sheet of paper black, but instead put up with the glaring colours. The best aspect about painting is the sensation of putting my hands into the wet paint in the pallet. This is a very unusual sensation. My hands feel surrounded and I can interact and be a part of this slippery wet paint. When the paint dries on my hands it makes them feel stiff and when I bend them the paint cracks, like the skin of an old person. For some inexplicable reason the Headmistress has told me that if I do not stop submerging my hands in the paint she will not allow me do any more paintings! Perhaps being an artist is not so desirable, since my father now says that even artists need to be able to read as they may have forms to fill in, bills to pay, etc.

When I grow up and need to read something, I will just have to ask someone to read it to me. I am unashamed of my inability to read because there are many other things I can do. My favourite topic is the universe. I already understand about the solar system and how the planets and moons move. I just wish that the earth's rotation did not make us all feel so dizzy. Maybe when I grow up I could become an astronaut and visit some galaxies or perhaps I could be an astronomer and learn about the universe. My father says if I want to be an astronaut or astronomer I will have to be excellent at maths, top of the class. Since I prefer astronomy to art I am going to make a huge effort to become brilliant at maths.

At home there is a small blackboard in my bedroom and recently I have often asked my father to write some sums on it for me to do. This is always risky because he always becomes cross when I get the answers wrong. Tonight is no exception. I have tried to do some adding sums and got them right but managed to make a mess of the subtraction. I do not understand the words '6 take away 2'.

"If you have 6 apples and I take 2 away how many do you have left?" asked my father. I really cannot comprehend what he is saying. I am unable to convert the words into a sensible array of pictures in my mind so he may as well be talking another language. I am having a flash of inspiration,

"Daddy, it does not matter whether I write '6-2' or '2-6' it will be the same".

"Do not be ridiculous, you cannot possibly have 2 apples and then take 6 away", he said in his irritated voice.

"But, Daddy", I tried to explain.

"Look, the sum 2-6 is impossible....", he said and then rattled on explaining the whole silly concept again. If only I could find the words to explain to him, that on an abstract level, the difference between 6-2 and 2-6 must surely and simply be the same. If he is correct and it is impossible to do the sum 2-6, the maths system we are using is a very strange system, which somehow bends back on itself, in other words is non-linear. This would be an over-complicated circular system. This experience led me to believe that everyone including the top adult scientists and mathematicians had got it wrong.

"Daddy, I do not need to go to school any more because I understand everything about maths", I exclaimed. He replied,

"I've never heard anything so ludicrous. You barely know anything. You are going to go to school and that is the end of the story." Perhaps, if I could understand the system of maths that everybody is using, maybe one day I will be able to explain my much better and simpler system. I spent weeks trying to imagine this bent and twisted system in which there was not a valid answer to the sum 2-6. After a few weeks I became so perplexed that I could not obtain the correct answer to any subtraction sum because I was unable to imagine the twisted system. Why do so many different things completely elude me?

Oh no, my mother is calling me,

"Yes, what do you want", I answered.

"Come down stairs, I want you to have another go at learning to read the time". Not again. Has she not realised that I am incapable of telling the time? After all, time has no meaning, so why would anyone need to be able to read a clock? My parents were sitting in the living room. Try and read the time from the clock face. Clocks faces are a complete mystery to me. I can never see which is the shorter hand nor can I tell which way round the hands move. In addition, the words 'quarter past', 'half past', 'quarter to' make no sense. It is the words 'past' and 'to' which confuse me, I cannot comprehend their meaning. So I will have to surmise what the time is. I think we may have had lunch, therefore it must be afternoon.

"Quarter past 3", I said guessing.

"Come on Alison you can do better than that. It is not the afternoon yet", said my father. Knowing that it is morning does not really help, because I really cannot make any sense out of a clock face. For ages we went round and round in circles. I kept guessing the time and my parents kept trying to teach me what to do. When I finally managed to escape from them, I still had no idea how to read the time and felt frustrated by the illusiveness of time. I think, my parents and the schoolteacher, probably perceive me as completely stupid. I hate school and all things to do with 'learning'.

'Home time' is my favourite time of day and once home, as always, I can investigate the world at large, at my leisure. Playtime is the other time of day when I am relatively free to do my investigating. Sometimes I run straight into the fence or ride my bike into stationary objects to see how it feels. Periodically I rush around and jump on people to see how they react. Now and then I shout until my throat is sore. However, most of my time is taken up with learning how to manipulate the objects called friends, by finding out how they function. There are many things to do and many games to play! On the whole I am okay at predicting the anger of my friends, classmates and most importantly of the teacher. All I need to predict is when they are about to get cross, that is the only important aspect of anyone's behaviour. I do this by trial and error to see what sorts of things push them over the edge. Sometimes I purposely make them angry because they appear very different and even funny.

My self-esteem has taken a huge battering this school year. I do not tell my parents how my schoolteacher is destroying me because it is my fault for being so weak and slow. Why should I give them further reason to be ashamed of me? It is nearing the end of this diabolical year with this teacher who I think of as odious. I have just won the handwriting competition in my class. At last I have achieved something good, surely this will please the teacher.

Why is the teacher appearing to tell me that despite winning the competition, my handwriting is not as good as many of the other children's entries in my class? The teacher is even showing me examples of my classmates' handwriting entries. It does not make any sense! Why does she seem so upset that I won? If I won, surely my handwriting is the best, isn't it? What do I need to do in order to convince this teacher that I am not a complete failure? While I wrote my entry for the handwriting competition I made my whole body become rigid, gripped my pencil very hard and forced my arm and hand into writing as neatly as possible. I rested my head on my other hand to stop myself from feeling too dizzy and to help me control my eye movement. I tried to hold my eyes still and also closed them slightly to reduce the glare from the page. I used a bookmark so that I did not completely lose my place. Having braced myself, I methodically wrote down each letter and remembered to leave gaps between the words. As always, my hand and arm became very stiff and painful. By the time I had finished, my body, head and eyes ached. What more does the teacher want from me? All year I have been practising my handwriting in an effort to form the letters neatly, and so increase my chances of being able to read my own work. I will not let this teacher see how upset I am over her apparent criticism of my handwriting. I shall continue my policy of trying to control all my negative emotional responses so that this teacher and others like her do not know my weakness. The end of the school year cannot come quickly enough.

When my parents visited the school for an end of year chat with the teacher, unbeknown to me, they were also shown copies of other children's entries into the handwriting competition and the teacher intimated that these other specimens were better than my entry. The end of year school report does not indicate any of my problems, not even the fact that my reading was appalling. I received a 'satisfactory' in all areas including reading and written English. I think the report was a farce, its overriding comment was 'She doesn't always find it easy but she tries hard and has made progress'! However, my parents knew there was something amiss because my sister who was 3 years younger was not experiencing the same problems with reading or writing and neither were my peer group. The burning question was; is Alison stupid or perhaps Dyslexic?

3

....Second Year Junior School (I was aged 9 for most of this academic year)....As my birthday is at the beginning of the academic year I was moved into a class which mostly contained children who were one academic year ahead (i.e. 3rd year juniors) of me. This was to work in my favour, for being one of the youngest in the class rather than one of the eldest, meant the teacher did not expect as much from me and was therefore more tolerant. This also meant that for the majority of the time I was free to investigate my environment at my leisure. At this stage I could do some maths to a reasonable level for my age, but was still unable to read.

I am greatly relieved that the teacher I had last academic year has definitely left the school and therefore she will never again be able to hurt me. I have used my skills for studying people and this year's teacher seems much softer and more pleasant, hopefully she will stay like this. She is of course like most teachers and indeed most people, in that she speaks mainly in garbled incomprehensible noises. In this class are two of my friends who live in the same street as I do. This gives me an acceptable sense of security. They are my reference points.

Often we have writing lessons. I have many ideas locked away in my wordless mind, but even when I find words that, at best, only partially express my thoughts, I have great difficulty in writing them down, because my spelling is extremely poor and my punctuation none existent. However, myself, the teacher and a friend, have found a mutually good solution. When I have finished a piece of work, I tell my friend what the words are supposed to say and she then corrects the majority of my spelling errors. This means the teacher is much more able to read what I have written and has to spend much less time deciphering my work. Consequently this takes the pressure off both the teacher and myself, plus my friend seems to enjoy helping me because she wishes to become a teacher (an ambition she was to fulfil).

This teacher is much more patient with me. When I go and read to her she does not shout, but rather, tries to encourage me. This is in stark contrast to my parents.

"Alison I've brought 2 books home for you to read", said my father as he came in from work.

"What are they about?" I asked.

"You will have to read them to find out", answered my father. Examination of the pictures within the book indicates to me that one of the books is about glass and glass making and the other is about cars.

"Alison, don't just look at the pictures, you must read the words", shouted my father across the room as he walked away. I asked,

"Mummy, please can you read these books to me?".

"No", booms my father. He continues, "You are to read the books yourself. Don't be so lazy. You will never learn to read if you do not practise. Go and sit in the lounge and read one of the books". As I look at the words in the book about glass making I cannot read enough of them to make any sense of it, which means I am going to have to ask what some of these words are. So I went over to my mother and asked,

"What do these words say?", while pointing at the page.

"Alison, I've told you that if you are going to learn to read you'll have to practise. Practise makes perfect. You are not going outside to play until you have read that book", roared my father. In despair I look at the words once again. What do the words say? I will just have to pretend to read the book! After sitting in the chair quietly for a while I leapt up saying,

"I've finished" and ran outside to the place where my friends were playing. Why do my parents think that giving me a book will solve all my reading problems? If I cannot read, confronting me with a book full of words I am unable to read is hardly going to help, particularly if nobody assists me!

My parents are full of strange ideas.

"Alison, your friends enjoy reading. They often do some reading on their own. Wouldn't it be a good idea if you became like them? If you do some reading on your own you will enjoy it", commented my mother. I do not understand how my friends can possibly enjoy reading. After all, it is clearly so painful. Reading obviously results in a headache as well as sore, achy eyes. In an effort not to lose my place, even my hands become sore because I use a bookmark to prevent myself from skipping lines and follow the letters with my finger so that they are not missed. How do people cope with the pain? Am I just a weak person less able to cope? It would be a mistake to admit to my parents how much trouble I have coping with the pain, because they will then realise how feeble I am and be even more disappointed in me.

At school today we have to do a word search through the dictionary. We must work in pairs and look up the meaning of a list of words. The whole exercise seems completely pointless for I cannot read the words or their explanations. My partner is much quicker than I am. He is looking up the words and writing down the answers before I have a chance to see any of the words on the page. Although I have tried to slow him down he insists that I just copy his answers. This would be fine except I cannot see or read what he has written! My only option is to try and write down something sensible.

It's not fair. I've tried so hard. The teacher has told me to redo the exercise because I have made a mess of it. But, it is nearly impossible to find a word in a dictionary, because I do not know the order of the alphabet. As I try to find some of the words in the dictionary my eyes become so tired. What is the point of doing something, which is so exhausting and painful? I have decided not to redo this exercise but instead to spend the rest of the afternoon talking to my friends, but never listening!

I try to do as little of the written work as possible, because when writing for more than a couple of minutes my arm starts to ache and becomes increasingly painful. In addition, my legs and non-writing arm start to ache, particularly when tracing or writing for long periods of time (e.g. Handwriting lessons). It is so hard to form letters so that they can be read by anybody, including myself. How do my friends manage to put up with this horrid pain? They do not complain, so I will put on a brave face and not complain either. I have no desire to appear weak. This means that when we are set tasks such as projects to do, I produce a few pages of writing and drawings, while others produce many pages. I never seem to get into trouble, so why bother to do more?

Friday comes around all too quickly. It is my worst day of the week because we have spelling tests. I never manage to learn the spellings and even if I manage to remember the sequence of letters for one or two of the words long enough to write them down in the test, the meaningless sequence of letters is soon forgotten. Often my mark is as low as, zero out of ten. The worst aspect is that we have to write out correctly 10 times, each spelling we get wrong. One of my friends has suggested that the best and quickest way to do this is to write the first letter of the word 10 times down the page, then the second and so on until the end of the word. Having tried this it is obvious that this is indeed the most efficient way of completing the spelling corrections! If the teacher catches me doing this I am sure she will be furious!

Things are becoming steadily worse at home. Jenny is learning to read. She can already read much better than myself despite being 3 years younger and having completed only one year at school. This is embarrassing and deeply frustrating because there is nothing I can do about it. If I am not careful my stupidity will become as apparent to Jenny as it is to my parents, teachers and many of my peer group. It is therefore important for me to try and prevent Jenny from realising that my reading is worse than hers is. I do not wish Jenny to realise my slowness and weakness. I wish I could be clever. In fairy tales Owls are supposed to be very wise. I wish I could become wise like the Owls in the fairy tales. If only I was not so stupid.

To make matters even worse at home, I have to work really hard at trying to keep ahead of Jenny in all areas of life, including sporty activities. I persevere with things like hitting, throwing and bouncing a ball as well as running, jumping, etc. so that Jenny does not show me up and to give myself a chance of competing with my friends. I often practise with great determination for hours on end. It does not matter how many times I have to hit or bounce that ball. I do not really know where my hand is in relation to the rest of my body, let alone the position of the flying ball. But somehow I will learn to control the ball. In addition, Jenny seems to have a much better relationship with my parents. It seems to be me who is always in trouble. If only I could be more like Jenny. However, at the moment I am so frustrated by my own weaknesses, that I am unable to feel friendly towards Jenny.

My parents smack and threaten me when I do not do the things they want me to do. Likewise if one of my friends, sister or classmates does not do what I wish them to do, I threaten and hit them. Besides, that is not my real mother anyway, she disappeared ages ago - didn't she? The impostor has never slipped up, so consequently nobody seems to have noticed her intrusion.

Each week I have to go to 'Brownies' (a section of the Girl Guides). Here I can get away with more-or-less anything. The other children who go to Brownies are all very clever, they can read, write, hear, remember etc. We are always being asked to do activities, which are far beyond me. For instance, tying knots, sewing, writing, catching balls and running. I am just so slow at everything. I spend the vast majority of the time messing around and being thoroughly silly; tickling my friend, turning off the hall lights, washing my hands in glue!, etc. Doing these things helps cover up for my inadequacies.

I do not want anyone, including my family or friends, to notice my lack of intelligence. One of my relatives said,

"Alison, tell me what the time is". I do not wish to reveal that I am still unable tell the time, therefore I shall give a daft answer,

"Tea Time!"

"Go on, read the time from the clock", my relative said. My relative can clearly see the clock, so why should I read the time? There is no need. I feel like an animal in the circus being asked to perform. I refuse to let anyone in on my secret,

"Lunch Time!"

"Alison, can you not be sensible for one moment?" replied the relative.

"No", I replied and ran off. Playing the fool is the easiest way to hide all the things I cannot do!

"Alison, show Jenny which is your left arm", demanded my relative. Does this person never let up? I do not exist for the amusement of others. Despite being told many times, I have no idea which is my left arm and which is the right. After all, both arms look exactly the same to me! Anyway who cares? Why give the arms separate names when they are the same. Again, I will have to play the fool and pretend to purposely get it wrong. My relative is becoming evermore frustrated and irritated by my apparent messing around. I prefer people to become cross rather than realise my shortcomings.

My 'Tick-tock' Nana[3] is a completely different story. She is wonderful. 'Tick-tock' Nana treats me like a normal human being and sticks up for me in front of my father. To her I am really special and she calls me her 'Best Girl', she makes me feel worth something. 'Tick-tock' Nana has my utmost respect, a respect which the rest of my family, friends, teachers, acquaintances, lost a long time ago. She treats me so well, so consequently I never mess her around and always treat her the best I know how. 'Tick-tock' Nana does not care if I cannot read, write, tell the time, etc. She considers that I am very intelligent, but most of all she believes in me.

At school, I am at last allowed to have a go at playing a musical instrument - the Recorder. It is hard for me to see which note is which, because they are just black blurs in amongst wiggly lines. It is also very hard for me to make my fingers open out far enough for them to go over the holes on the recorder. However, I can mostly see whether the next note is higher or lower relative to the one being played. Unbeknown to me, my parents were surprised that I was managing to learn to play the recorder, since they thought I would never manage to master reading music if reading words were too difficult!

There is some indication on the report that I have trouble reading and writing. For Reading, Writing and Maths I was awarded a minus. In all other areas received a 'satisfactory'. In the maths section the teacher has commented 'Alison can produce good work if she has grasped the initial method, however she is sometimes slow to do this'. This is hardly surprising considering I was trying to conceptualise a twisted mathematical system, which did not contain negative numbers! Worse still, by this time we were learning about division and again I was soon sure there was a valid answer to a division sum, whichever way the numbers were divided. Unfortunately, I had no way of proving it and when told that I was wrong, I became even more convinced that the system of maths that everyone was using was very cumbersome and twisted. On the school report the teachers overall comment was 'Alison tries hard but needs to concentrate more fully on the task in hand'. I did not comprehend the concept of 'concentration'!

---

[3] As a child this was the name I gave to my paternal grandmother and will continue to use it throughout this book.

4

This summer holiday I am going with Shirley Nana to stay with a relation, Edna, who I barely know. Shirley Nana is an acceptable reference point and my main concern is what food we will be given to eat. Will there be anything I like to eat? Will I starve? My mother says Edna eats normal food but I am unconvinced. Despite Shirley Nana being an acceptable reference, I feel extremely terrified as we leave the station on the train. It is important to me that she does not see my weakness and fear because she would probably think I was daft. I feel terrible as we stop at the stations. I know that the train is stationary but as I look out of the window the station seems to be moving all over the place, often it looks and feels as if the train is still moving forward. After what seemed like an extraordinary amount of time we arrived at our destination. As we got off the train, for some completely inexplicable reason, Edna and my grandma threw their arms around each other, after which we were taken by car to Edna's house.

"k afo we$^{a\wedge}$ofn wk#fk,ewjflfnl*WEFH", said Edna. I am accustomed to having terrible trouble understanding what people say, but this is ridiculous. Is she even speaking English?! This is awful. I have arrived in a strange house and the only person I can mostly understand is Shirley Nana. I feel so alone and scared, they must not see my tears. This emotional response must be quashed, NOW.

"Oh dear, Alison has gone all silly and shy. Come on Alison, reply to Edna's question", said Shirley Nana. Well, I would answer if I had any idea what she may have just garbled. How does Shirley Nana understand Edna?

Having been here a few hours, I am beginning to adapt to this strange accent and to understand some of the words Edna and her family are saying. It appears that Edna does speak English but has a very strong accent (In retrospect, I now appreciate that Edna's accent is not broad and is relatively similar to mine!). I soon realised that Edna was a really great person just like my 'Tick-tock' Nana. Edna has told me some very interesting facts about myself. She tells me, that I have much more trouble remembering many things than other people do and that I forget many things really quickly. This is very odd because I had believed that my memory was excellent, but I can now see what she means. Edna also tells me that I tend to get things back to front and mixed up round the wrong way much more than most people. Is this the real reason why I do so badly at school? For the first time in my life I realise that something is amiss. It is a relief to know that there are some good reasons for my poor performance at school. Maybe I am not stupid after all. Perhaps Edna was unaware that I had no idea that other people do not have these problems. In case this is true I will be very careful how I ask my mother about my problems when we return home. I do not wish to get Edna into trouble because she has been so good to me and it would be great if we could come and see her again in the future. It makes me so angry to think that my parents never bothered to tell me about my problems. They obviously do not care about me. Or does Edna understand more about me than they do?

5

....Third Year Junior School (I was aged 10 for most of this academic year)....Since my birthday is at the beginning of the academic year I was again put into a class which mostly contained children who were one academic year ahead (i.e. final year juniors) of me. Despite being one of the youngest in the class the teacher still expected me to behave in a more mature fashion and to do much of the same work as the older children. My parents became ever more concerned over my lack of progress with reading and writing and became increasingly convinced that Dyslexia was my problem. They were perplexed. One moment I was building a complex Lego model without any instructions, or building something I had seen being made on a Children's T.V. programme and ingeniously improvising for the parts which were not readily available in our home. But in the next moment I was unable to do the simplest of tasks properly, for instance, retrieving an object from upstairs without forgetting what I was supposed to be doing before I had reached the top of the stairs. Or I would lay the table for dinner with some of the knives and forks on the wrong sides of the place mats (our family all eat the right-handed way). My parents wondered, is Alison unintelligent? Or is Alison just lazy? Or both?

I am becoming fairly good at quashing all my emotional fears and try very hard to convince myself that nothing whatsoever scares me. This seems the best way to overcome my fears of the chaotic bedlam in which we all live. However, I really do not understand how other people manage to control their fears of our manic environment in an apparently effortless way. It is my first day in this class and already I have been in trouble twice, initially for chatting and then for crawling across the floor to the other side of the room. My intention was to reach my destination without being seen by the teacher! Am I losing my touch? Maybe I had better spend a few days sizing up this teacher and finding out where his weak points lie. The classroom is as visually and audibly manic as all other public places and the teacher talks in fragmented sounds and expects us to understand him. Why do so many people have voices that are hard to understand? It is much easier to understand voices that I often hear such as, those of my parents, sister and long standing friends, but unfamiliar voices are very hard to master. Everybody seems to speak so differently.

I do not know why the teacher wishes my desk to be so close to his. It makes it much harder for me to do what I like without getting into trouble. The other bad aspect about the position of my desk is that the blackboard is behind me, on my left side (i.e. when sitting at my desk my back faces towards the blackboard). When copying from the blackboard I cannot keep twisting my head around to see the blackboard as this obviously makes me feel very dizzy and is excruciatingly painful to my neck. The only other alternative is to slide across the surface of the chair so that my body faces the blackboard, but I soon become dizzy and disorientated. This makes copying anything from the blackboard very hard, but despite these obvious problems I am often told off for being careless. Does the teacher not realise how hard I try?

For about the last year I have been developing a way of remembering exactly where my eyes are on a page of writing or on a blackboard. This is clearly needed if a person is to quickly copy anything onto a separate sheet of paper. My friends have already perfected this and I have been stupidly slow in realising that this is required. First I look at the blackboard, at the place I am up to. Then I read a few more letters, remember exactly how my eye muscles feel at the place I have got up to, keep my body rigid so that it remains still, then I look down to my page and write down the next few letters. Finally I look back at the blackboard, recall how my eye muscles felt and make my muscles go back to that position. However, my new strategy does not work very well when the blackboard is behind me!

The teacher hollered,

"For goodness sake stop yawning Jack." The only reason people yawn is to express their boredom or sometimes their tiredness. It is curious I am unable to work out how it is done! Whenever I try to imitate someone yawn it always comes out wrong. Hopefully I can soon find out how to yawn and then I will be able to express my true boredom.

When I cannot do the work we are presented with, or become bored, I often stare at the billions and billions of infinitesimally small bits, which zoom around randomly across everything we all, see. These strange and curious minute bits are always present and are of course very prominent across the brightness of the sky. When I look at a page of writing, the bits often appear to form rivers, which flow between the words. What are these bits? What are they made of?

At night the billions of bits are most annoying. No matter how dark it is in a room, I can still see the bits manically dancing around all over everything. I am sure they would be invisible if only my room could be made completely dark. The bits can become even wilder when I close my eyes. They form into groups of colour, which move around in and out of my vision growing and shrinking in size while varying in shape. When I am lying in bed trying to go to sleep, these random, uncontrollable patterns can cause me to feel very dizzy and disorientated. I have the sensation of floating around the room. These are not dreams or thoughts from my imagination since I can still visualise objects in my mind in the normal way. The patterns are always there, when I close my eyes at night, when I wake up in the morning and at all other times during the day, including when I close my eyes. So what are these bits and patterns that I actually see? I have asked but nobody ever seems to understand what I am talking about, probably because I do not know how to express myself properly. Maybe one day in the future I will discover what they are.

Liquid Crystal display (LCD) Digital Watches have just come into the shops and are all the rage. Maybe, I would be able to read this type of clock face? After all, I can read figures. If I can persuade someone to buy me a digital watch it might solve all my problems with being unable to read the time. Having nagged my parents sufficiently about digital watches I have finally received a digital watch as a Christmas present from my grandparents. I have very quickly become accustomed to reading the numbers and can now finally hide, without playing the fool, the fact that I cannot read an analogue clock face. The main problem with the digital watch is that I cannot tell the difference between a 2 and a 5 because they are symmetrical, they look the same. I shall wear the watch all the time and perhaps, it will help me come to terms with the mysterious thing called time.

Now that I can read the time, I know when it is lunch break and no longer need to watch the other children to see if I should be taking my lunch out of my bag. On many an embarrassing occasion in the past I have thought either, it was lunch in our first break, did not realise it was the lunch break, or thought someone had stolen all my food in the break after lunch! (When I had already eaten it.)

Oh dear, what a shame! Yet again I am going to miss PE! (physical education i.e. sports) Today, instead of being humiliated in a PE lesson I have to go and have remedial English lessons to help me with my reading and writing. The remedial teacher drones on and on, in a voice I can hardly understand and asks me to do babyish things. Why should I listen to this woman? I think it is very dumb of the remedial teacher to expect me to do homework. I never do it!

"What are you doing standing out here?", asked the headmistress. So I replied,

"I am waiting for the remedial English teacher. My lesson is now in school assembly time, so that I do not miss PE or anything else." I did not realise up until now, but the headmistress is aware that I never do any homework. She is asking to see it.

"I have not done any homework." I answered proudly. The headmistress went red in the face and asked me how I expected to improve. She then continued to sternly tell me that the remedial lessons were for my benefit and that I should always do the homework. I have been told to do last week's homework while waiting for the remedial teacher to arrive. The headmistress stormed off to the morning Assembly. My friends do not have extra English homework, so why should I? Still, there would be no harm in doing it while I wait, I suppose. There is nowhere for me to sit so I will have to kneel down and rest my work on a narrow bench. A while later, after I had finished my homework, the headmistress reappeared and demanded to know whether I had done the homework. Then proceeded to firmly tell me that if she ever again heard that I was not doing my homework, I would be in big trouble and my mother would be told. I think the headmistress is a nasty person. Why does the headmistress think that threatening me will make me do the pointless homework? After all, I need not tell my mother that I have homework. Having finished the remedial lesson, I returned to my usual class to discover, to my horror, the headmistress was filling in for our normal teacher, who is off sick.

Why me? I am already in trouble and I have barely stepped inside the classroom. The headmistress wants me to go over to her desk. At least she is no longer shouting at me. Dragging my feet I negotiated the cluttered desks and reluctantly went over to her desk. Excellent, she says that the cover design I did for the forthcoming school play programme was the best out of all those, which were submitted. She continued by saying that she was still very cross with me for failing to do my homework and that she did not feel that I deserved my design to go on the front cover of the programme. But despite this she has decided that my design is the best and therefore it will go on the front cover. Perhaps my low opinion of the headmistress is not justified, because although she is cross with me, she is still prepared to put my design on the front cover. This impresses me. She has won a minute amount of my respect.

The cover design was for a play, set in a 19th Century coffee house in Istanbul and depicted a wood seller's changing fortunes.

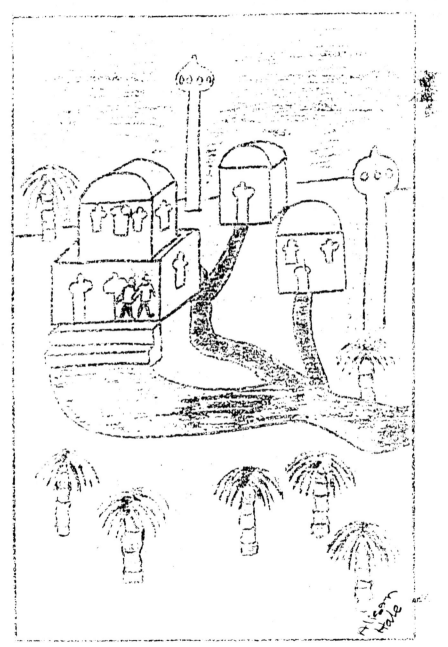

My mother has allowed me to start having piano lessons, since I have been able to keep up with the Recorder lessons at school. The idea of learning to play the piano is particularly attractive because this is an opportunity that Jenny and most of my friends do not have. Consequently there is no pressure of performing to a certain standard within a set time scale. The down side is that piano playing is so painful on my hands, arms and especially my shoulders. This must be the price all pianists pay for making their fingers press down the keys. I have no idea how anyone manages to open his or her adjacent fingers out so that each finger can be placed over a separate key. The most logical way around this problem seems to be, to first teach myself how to open the fingers on one hand whilst using the other hand to force the fingers apart. Then to swap hands and in the same way teach myself to open the fingers on the other hand.

After much practise I have had some limited success. Maybe, eventually my fingers will open up properly of their own accord. I really cannot imagine how anyone manages to read two staves (lines) of music at once (left and right hand), for it is obvious that, nobody can possibly see both staves at the same time! After all, it is only possible to see one note simultaneously and therefore infeasible to see a note which is on the stave below. The obvious simple solution must be to memorise the music from one of the staves and read the other. I wish piano playing were not so tiring.

I seem to tire more quickly than my friends do. How can I overcome this? It is important to me that nobody knows my weakness, after all, I wish to appear normal. The obvious solution seems to be for me to conserve my energy. To achieve this I will have to be as efficient as possible in the way I use my body. Consequently, I shall endeavour not to do too many unnecessary physical actions i.e. I will use my brain before my body. From now on I will always take the shortest routes in all my physical actions and academic work. For instance, walk the shortest amount of distance and miss out superfluous stages in all things.

In addition, to combat the tiredness I should try to go off to sleep quicker rather than lying awake for ages engulfed in weird sensations. I have deduced that to go off to sleep quicker I must stop my mind from thinking. In other words, clear my mind of all thoughts, since when we are asleep we do not think. So every night I lie down in bed and keep throwing away all the thoughts that come into my mind. This seems to be a hard thing to master, but I believe that when mastered my problems with going to sleep will end.

It is now a long time since I visited Edna and a convenient moment for me to quiz my mother about my memory and reversal problems.

"Mummy, I seem to forget things quicker than other people and get things back to front more often", I casually commented. My mother agreed and started telling me a bit more about my problems. It is a great weight off my mind to know that my inability to read is at least partly explainable. My mother tells me there is no cure for my problems and that I will have to work hard to overcome them. This does not sound too good! Thankfully Edna alerted me to the fact that I am not totally stupid or a complete failure. When would my mother have bothered to tell me? Probably never. Perhaps my parents wanted me to think of myself as unintelligent.

My parents are always expecting me to set a good example to Jenny. If I do something wrong and get caught by my parents, I of course receive a smack, but if Jenny happens to have copied my naughty act she does not get into trouble. Jenny says to my parents,

"Alison is the eldest, she should set me a good example". Usually this does the trick and she either gets into no trouble or considerably less trouble. I feel that my parents are always substantially more tolerant towards her behaviour just because she is younger. Can Jenny not be accountable for her own actions? Why should I carry the burden of responsibility for her behaviour? Another thing, which really irritates me, is when my parents allow Jenny to do activities that I was not allowed to do at her age. It is hard enough staying ahead of her without my parents giving her an unfair start. Do my parents purposely do this in the hope that Jenny will overtake me and show me up? I have become very frustrated with Jenny for causing me so many extra hassles. Since my parents treat Jenny in a more tolerant way they obviously prefer her, but why? Maybe I am adopted? Yes, I must be adopted, that would explain many things. Or perhaps the intruder, who calls herself my mother, has taken a dislike to me. Since my parents are not fond of me, will they send me to boarding school? Boarding school would remove me out of their way. Perhaps I should just run away? Where would I go? To 'Tick-tock' Nana's flat? To Edna's house? It feels like nobody understands anything about me.

As the year has progressed my friends who are an academic year ahead of me have matured and grown far beyond me. There seems to be no way of bridging the gap and balancing out things again. They have abandoned me and I have been left to play with the children who are my age in the class. Will things ever return to the way they were? I miss them because they were a large part of my reference system. I am dreading next academic year because they will not even be at this school. I will be alone.

In my end of year report I received a minus in reading, written English & mathematics. Under written English the teacher wrote 'Much of her written work is good but suffers from lapses'. Under Mathematics the teacher wrote 'She finds some difficulty in this work but she works hard. She is more confident when solving practical problems'. This was usually because I could not understand the English used to describe abstract problems. The overall comment was 'Alison has made progress during the year. Mostly she works hard but is inclined to gossip unless close attention is given. She possesses drive and could make very positive progress if she put her mind to it.' My parents were annoyed that I had spent yet another year in a class full of children older than myself. They felt that the teacher's main concern was preparing the older children for secondary school and not worrying about my lack of progress, because I still had one more year at primary school to complete.

6

....Fourth Year Junior School (I was aged 11 for most of this academic year)...The further I went through my education the more my English skills fell behind. This was obviously of great concern to my parents. Unbeknown to me they had been to see the headmistress to voice their concerns. At this point the headmistress appeared to feel that I was just a slow learner and if I had enough intelligence I would eventually catch up. My parents had for several years, been trying to help me to learn some basic phonetics and then to use this knowledge to help with spelling. The headmistress was to teach my class for the whole of the final year.

I have all the usual reservations about being in this class: manic noise, chaotic visual environment, finding stable references (e.g. desk, coat hook, etc), teacher's personality, and the attitudes of fellow classmates. The teacher knows very little about me and I am sure most of it is unfavourable, so she will probably treat me badly. I will observe her weaknesses. However, she always praises my art work. My mother and grandfather have given me much help in learning to draw objects in the conventional way. They both say I should draw exactly what I see, but the style they are teaching me does not incorporate the fuzziness or all the bits flying around. This seems contradictory. Everything must be straight and clear with the correct foreshortening. (In hindsight, I learnt to draw so that my drawings appeared normal, but they were not a true reflection of what I actually saw. My great desire and determination, to be 'normal' and good at drawing, hid my visual problems.)

During a science lesson the teacher claimed that a straight line is made up of a series of curves and if we could look at a straight line that was extremely long, we would be able to see its curvature. I would have thought that this was obvious. As I sit here looking across the classroom at the walls, ceiling and blackboard, they all appear to be very slightly curved. The only straight lines which do not appear curved are those which are relatively very short e.g. a 10 millimetre (0.4 inch) line. It is really very strange what most teachers decide to teach us. They must assume we are all incapable of observing and reasoning for ourselves.

The teacher keeps telling me that when I read I should stop screwing up my face because there is no need and it does not look very good. But, if I try not to screw up my face the paper appears even brighter and it is much harder to control my eyes. Screwing up my face aids me in controlling the movement of my eyes, which in turn makes more letters clearer, so enabling me to follow the letters more accurately, thus improving my reading. Since everybody does this, why shouldn't I?

Later, I said to my mother,

"I am having trouble reading this book because the writing is too small".

"Alison, I've never in all my life, heard such a ridiculous excuse for not reading.", replied my mother in an irritated voice. I had better explain myself,

"It's true! The smaller the writing, the harder it is to read".

"I've never heard anything so completely ludicrous", said my father. He continued, "The only reason you like books with big writing is because they have more pictures. Looking at pictures won't help you learn to read."

"But Daddy, I don't care about the pictures. I am just trying to say how much more difficult it is to read small writing.", I replied.

"It is no good trying to make such silly excuses, because you'll never learn to read. You are your own worst enemy." My father is obviously talking nonsense. He must know that it is harder to read smaller writing. Why does he say these silly things? Does he think I am so dense that I will believe him?

"Mummy, I always get a headache when I read", I commented.

"Do not make such daft excuses. You do not get a headache from reading", replied my mother in a cross manner. Now my mother is also talking nonsense. She must know that everybody gets headaches from reading. Clearly, I must be much worse at coping with the pain than other people, so I will refrain from making further comments, as I do not wish my parents to become even more ashamed of me. So I continued trying to read. When Shirley Nana came into the room, she heard me trying to read and asked,

"Can Alison see properly?"

"She has been to the opticians recently and they said apart from being very slightly short-sighted, there is no problem with her eyesight. Why do you ask?", replied my mother.

"The thing that makes me wonder, is that when Alison reads she does not phrase what she is reading, there is no expression", answered Shirley Nana who continued by saying, "She reads in a monotone." My mother replied,

"Oh, that's nothing to do with being unable to see properly. It is because she barely has the reading age of a 7-year-old. Children who are 7 years old do not phrase what they are reading, particularly if they hesitate the way Alison does."

"I see the same as everybody else", I commented. (At the time, I had no frame of reference other than myself, therefore did not realise that I saw differently to anybody else, consequently I was unable to verbalise my unusual perceptions.)

I can hear my mother speaking on the phone,

".....Jenny is doing fine at school. Yes, she is about average. I think that if she put her mind to it she could do a little better. Alison... well, she is still struggling on". Can my mother not say anything about how good I am at practical things? Why does everybody judge me on my lack of academic progress? What is wrong with saying things about practical work? Who can say which are more important, academic or practical things? Reading and writing are not the only things in life. My mother continues speaking,

"......she tries hard, but does not seem to be making much progress." What does she expect me to do, draw blood? Sometimes this can literally be the case. I get so frustrated that I tear bits of skin off my fingers. Why does my mother have to implicitly mention how weak I am at coping with the pain? My mother continues her conversation,

"......Yes, I think she is probably Dyslexic. When she is reading she perceives all the words mixed up, but I am not sure how!" What is my mother talking about now? I see just like everybody else!

It sometimes takes me ages to start a piece of written work because I do not know which side of the piece of paper to begin, or which way to move my hand across the paper. However, if I do actually start I am fine. One aspect of Christmas that I really loath is writing thank you letters. So that I do not show my parents up, I struggle for ages trying to write something sensible, but whatever I write, it is never good enough.

"Come on Alison this is not good enough, you have written this letter like a 7 year old", says my mother as she struggles to read my spelling. Demoralised, I return to my room to have another attempt. By the time I return with a modified letter Jenny has also written a draft of her letter. My mother corrects my spelling then reads aloud the letter. She reads it in a staccato, monotone style as if what I have written is completely useless. To make matters even worse she then proceeds to read Jenny's letter fluently. Why does my mother have to show up my English in front of Jenny? Why could she not have read both our letters fluently? Surely, my letter is not that bad?

In creative writing I like to write stories about terrible disasters, because I would like to know how I would cope in such situations and how my family would react. Often I kill off my mother, father, more often than not Jenny and have even killed off myself. This allows me to explore the possibilities of any member of my family no longer being around, since I like the idea of getting rid of all the tension between the members of my family and myself. Jenny hurts me so much by being more favoured by my parents and my parents hurt me by not accepting me the way I am.

I commented to the teacher,

"Wouldn't it be funny if we had a fire in the school." I want to know how she would react under an emergency situation like a fire. I did not literally mean a fire would be 'funny', but my lack of eloquence prevents me from fully expressing myself. I really mean it would be fascinating. The strangeness of her reply intrigues me because she seems to think that it would not be and people could get hurt. Why should I care if the objects called people get hurt, or even die? Besides, if there were fewer children at the school there would be less chaos and that would be better for those who survived. Having thought a little more a better idea has come to me so I said,

"If the school was burnt down, we wouldn't have to come here any more".

The teacher reply is quite worrying because she seems to think that I would then have to go to school somewhere else". I guess this is true, but going to another school is definitely a bad idea.

"They wouldn't send our class to another school because we will soon be going off to the secondary school. Jenny might get killed", I said joyfully. The teacher's reply is very perplexing. She seems concerned and appears to think that I do not really mean that it would literally be good if Jenny died. I guess I better not disappoint the teacher. So I said, lying,

"Well, I suppose it would not be good if Jenny died". The teacher does not realise how much less pressure there would be on me if Jenny were not around. Without Jenny at home my parents would have to appreciate me more.

As we were taken home from school in a friend's mother's car, the mother explained why she had been late collecting us,

"There was a bad car crash on the road which was causing congestion, several cars were smashed."

"Wow! I wish I'd seen the accident", I exclaimed.

"I don't think you mean that," said the mother. I think she is wrong. It would be fascinating to see an accident and see how the cars crumple in a collision. It would also be interesting to see what happens to the people inside the cars. So I asked my friend's mother,

"Was there blood all over the road? Were there dead people in the road?" The other children in the car are screaming at my questions and my friend's mother is cringing. Why are they reacting like this to a perfectly reasonable enquiry? My friends have a very peculiar way of behaving.

Before entering this academic year I only had one or two friends at a time. This was easier for me to cope with for several reasons. When in a crowd of people, I am unable to process and make sense of all their movements and sounds. I really do not know how other people can process all this chaos. Therefore when faced with only a couple of people I usually understand at least some of what they are saying and doing. This year, I am finding it difficult, a few of my classmates are okay, but most of them are fairly bitchy for much of the time. I cannot be bothered to waste my precious energy on such silly, awkward behaviour. Most of the children hold no interest for me and therefore I do not wish to interact with them.

My idol is Mr. Spock from the television series Star Trek. He follows the doctrine of the people on his home planet. He uses logic to understand and interpret the world and has quashed all his emotional responses. I also use logic to understand the world. I am no different from everyone else; often emotions appear from nowhere and normally without any apparent reason. All I need to do is to ignore the emotions and concentrate on extending my logical analysis of the world just like Mr. Spock. Doing this should make me a better person. This is obviously the doctrine that everybody in the future will follow. Why does everybody seem so blind to its advantages?

At bedtime, I am still perfecting my method for going off to sleep by emptying all the thoughts from my mind. The method of focusing my mind on nothing really seems to be working. I have now had some inspiration for solving yet another night-time problem. I am fed up with persistently (several times a week) having nightmares, in which I fall off an object and as I crash to the ground wake up with a start. It has occurred to me that the best way to stop this is to wake myself up before I hit the ground, or preferably, just before I fall off the object. It is my aim to program my brain to wake me up in such nightmares. After a couple of initial failures I can now wake up and stop myself from crashing into the ground.

Unfortunately, this is not so easy in real life. I am always falling over, falling off things, falling into things and tripping over my clumsy feet! I need a better strategy for controlling myself so that these ungainly things happen less frequently. One answer is to stop turning my head, since turning it makes me dizzy and disorientated and therefore more liable to fall over. As I turn my head, things just blur past my eyes, I cannot see anything. If I can stop turning my head it should also stop me from continuously ricking my neck and thus reduce the pain. I am always looking for new strategies and consistency in the way 'the world' operates.

I have been experimenting with pocket calculators. Some calculators give an 'E' when a large number is subtracted from a small number, which implies there is no answer to such a sum. But others give the same figure as if the subtraction sum had been done around the other way. I am perplexed. They cannot both be correct and my father still insists, that subtracting a large number from a small one is an impossible sum. Also I have noticed that calculators will do division sums such as 1 divided by 100 and here again my father says this is impossible. Is the answer too complicated for my father to understand? What is going on? Who is stupid, my father, the calculator manufacturer's, or me?

My family are always expecting too much of me, but even more irritating is the response I get from so called 'friends of the family' such as Aunty Susan, Uncle John and their daughter Becky.

"Can't you tie shoe laces yet?" Uncle John said in a surprised mocking tone.

"What's that, Alison can't even do up shoelaces?!" said Aunty Susan. I wish they would leave me alone. Next time I will ask my mum to buy trainers that do not have laces, but instead use Velcro strips as fasteners. It is extremely hard to tie any type of knot. The words to describe how to tie knots never seem to make any sense; left over right, then right round behind left end, then through the loop.... My friends do not seem to have the same trouble as me. It is no help if someone shows me how to tie a knot, because I cannot see which piece goes where. I suppose I had better think up some defence,

"I am not very good at doing knots or bows. I don't usually have shoes which have laces in them."

"Becky has known how to tie shoelaces for years and when I was young we all knew how to............", replied Aunty Susan. Who cares what happened when she was young! I guess that Aunty Susan and Becky are like my friends, instantly good at everything, unlike me who is so slow. Why do these so-called 'friends of the family' emphasize my bad points?

I never know what my father is talking about when he tries to explain things. For instance, he has tried to teach me how to throw a 'Frisbee'. He demonstrates how to throw it, then tells me to do the same. I just do not know how to move my body to make it do the required task and am unable to copy the actions of other people. He puts the Frisbee in my hand and puts my arm in the starting position and then tells me to throw it. But despite being able to see which hand the Frisbee is in, there is no way for me to tell what action to make to throw it. I am even unsure which arm to move and in which direction. He grabs hold of my arm and forces it to make the correct movement but I have no idea how to repeat the movement. I cannot feel where any part of my body is in relation to the rest of my body and he moves my arm too quickly for me to literally 'see' and deduce what to do.

It is the same story whenever my father tries to show me how to do something. I always fail. He always treats me as if I am daft. Worse still is when we go bird watching. My father says to me,

"Look at the Yellowhammer in that tree".

"What tree" I answer.

"That one right in front of us" says my father.

"Which one" I reply. He points to where I should be looking.

"I still can't see which tree", I comment honestly. Finally my father grabs my head.

"Ouch!" He is disorientating me; I cannot process all this information. He turns my head into the correct position.

"I still can't see the Yellowhammer" I comment. He replies angrily,

"For goodness sake it is right in front of your nose! Open your eyes." I do of course have my eyes open but it does not seem to help! My father is always telling me to 'open my eyes' and that 'things are right in front of my nose'. I must be slow and useless in the way I use my eyes. So as usual I end up lying and saying,

"Oh yes, I see it." I always remember which birds we are supposed to have seen so that when we return home I can tell my mother which birds we have supposedly seen! I lie because I am so ashamed of my slowness and lack of intelligence also I do not wish my parents to realise the full extent of my inability because they would be even more ashamed of me.

Each summer it is the same. My father insists that Jenny and I 'top and tail' his home grown gooseberries ready for freezing. We have to sit out in the garden, each with a pair of small scissors and a bucket full of gooseberries. Cutting the tops and tails off the gooseberries is a very fiddly job, and causes pain in my head, eyes, neck, shoulders, arms, hands and legs. Why does he torture Jenny and myself in this way? Is my father vindictive? But the torture does not end there. My mother periodically retrieves some of the gooseberries from the freezer, stews and serves them up to be eaten. My parents insist that I should eat the gooseberries, despite my protesting and explaining that they are very painful to eat. When I put one in my mouth, excruciating pain shoots around the pivot area of my jawbones and partially seizes up my jaws. It then takes a huge amount of effort for me to actually bite and once bitten, the inside flesh of the gooseberry feels as if it is burning the inside of my mouth. After I have finished a bowl of gooseberries, my jaw still feels stiff and the inside of my mouth and tongue feel rough and very sore for many hours. Gooseberries are one of many fruits, which have this effect. (For example apples, pineapple and rhubarb also have this effect.) Why do people eat such painful food? Are they all mad? I try not to complain too much, for I am ashamed of my inability to endure the pain.

Success. Today, for the first time in my school life I have managed to obtain 100 house points for good work in an academic year. This means I become a 'Centurion'. For me, this is a great achievement. Most people in my class have accomplished this at least once sometime during their school life. As the day wears on I am beginning to regret rushing around madly in a celebratory mood, since I am now in so much extra pain as a result of this excitement. I received at least half of the house points for my practical work e.g. art, craft, designing and building. The teacher commented that I was a very practically minded person. Does this mean that even though I cannot read and write properly that I have good prospects for the future? Will I be able to become an artist, if I am never good enough at English and maths to become a scientist? Maybe there is some hope for my future. I have found that the older I become the greater peoples' expectations are of me. Will this always be the case?

I am anxious to go back inside to the safety of my classroom so I am waiting by the outside door until the bell is rung. Just as the bell rings my leg makes a sudden involuntary action and before I can stop my leg it flies straight into an empty milk bottle, shattering it into many pieces. Why does my body often make unintentional actions? The teacher will never believe me if I tell her what happened, nobody ever does under these circumstances. Hopefully, she will not realise that it was me who did this. The next day, still nothing had been mentioned about the broken bottle so I assumed she did not know who had broken it.

"Alison", I heard the teacher call. As I walked towards the playground. She grabbed me. What's happening to me? There are too many inputs from my body for my brain to process. Oh, it's okay. She has got her arm around my shoulders. But why? I must try and stay calm. She has now quietly asked me whether it was me who smashed the milk bottle yesterday afternoon. How could she have known it was me?

"Well......yes. It was me." I nervously answered. Now she wants to know how it happened and why I did not tell her. She is still talking quietly. Does this mean she is not angry? How am I going to explain this accident away!

"My foot just accidentally swung out and hit the bottle! Sorry", I replied. I do not know whether she ever believed my explanation. But strangely she never told me off. Why?

After spending two terms in her class, she had plenty of time to get to know me and began to wonder whether I was reasonably intelligent, based on the lateral thinking I was able to apply to practical tasks. To discover once and for all, she conducted a set of standard intelligence tests on me while the rest of the class was playing Rounders. The tests revealed that I had an IQ of good average intelligence, but barely had the reading age of an eight-year-old. The other confusing thing was that I did not exhibit the confusion, muddle or messiness the teacher expected to see in a 'true' Dyslexic. By this time the teacher could be fairly sure that I came from a stable family background and that there were no other apparent external factors for my inability to read. She spent a long time after school discussing with my mother the best way forward. One problem was nobody would officially say 'Alison has Dyslexia' since many still doubted the existence of the disorder.

A few weeks later a local expert who dealt with children with 'learning disabilities' is alleged to have told my mother that even if I was 'Dyslexic' there was nothing that could be done because I was now too old! (Retrospectively this is now known to be untrue, a Dyslexic person can be helped at any age.) My mother was recommended to take me through a book specially designed to help Dyslexic children learn to spell. Over the coming year she taught me all the phonetics anyone would ever want to know. For instance, spelling the word 'academic' is relatively simple because it is spelt the same way as it is pronounced i.e. ac - a - dem - ic. However, to spell words such as 'doubt' I must remember that the middle letters are 'ou' (as opposed to 'ow') and that there is a 'b' before the 't'. Once I had learnt all the phonetics in the English language and many of the rules and exceptions to the rules, I was in a much stronger position to read and spell. (Even today I still depend on the phonetics to enable me to read and spell. Someone once suggested that letter patterns correctly reached my brain but on the way out to my hand they became distorted, causing poor spelling.)

I had absolutely no perception of what to expect at secondary school, or any of the ramifications of leaving the primary school. I did not even realise that I would never return to the primary school as a pupil. As it came near to the time when we were due to leave I wrote the following about my life at the school.

Wednesday 15 July 8

I started this school the Mrs X..... in Mrs X..... every thing went wrong I never got eney English right
Wille I was in Mrs X..... When we were lining up to go to dinner I was standing next to Alison and then Mrs X..... palled me out of nay line and tood me to stop ginnering I was hot and I went back into the line after I had walked aa fuoo steps easat the same happan Mr X..... awer expands thing in mars bars in
This year I have ben in Mrs X..... class we have been campping for a week and don lots of thing I am looking fowd to my next school

The names have been deleted to maintain the anonymity of the people involved. For anyone who is not accustomed to reading a Dyslexic style of English and spelling this is what I wrote:-

> I started this school the Mrs X...*(last year infants)*.. In Mrs X...*(1st year juniors)*.. everything went wrong, I never got any English right. While I was in Mrs X...*(2nd year juniors)*.. when we were lining up to go to dinner I was standing next to ...*a friend*.. and then Mrs X...*(dinner lady)*.. pulled me out of my line and told me to stop grinning, I was not and I went back into the line. After I had walked a few steps exactly the same thing happened. Mr X...*(3rd year juniors)*.. always explains things in Mars Bars. In this year I have been in Mrs X...*(4th year juniors)*.. class we have been camping for a week and done lots of things. I am looking forward to my next school.

To me, my handwriting looks messy. This was my neatest and had I written less neatly, would have been unable to read my own work. I wrote 'I am looking forward to the next school', since that was what I thought we were supposed to write. What I really felt was the deepest fear and dread imaginable because I could not envisage any aspect of secondary school life. All I could imagine was a void in which all the rules of conduct were unknown. What would happen at lunch time? How would I conduct myself? How would I speak to people? How would I find my way around? This was terrifying, because I could not imagine ever having the answers.

At the end of the year, the teacher indicated to me her feelings on my progress and wrote them in the end of year report. This report was perhaps the most honest I had received up to this point in my school life. I received a minus for reading, with the comment 'Alison is deserving of great praise for her efforts to overcome severe difficulties. She should not be discouraged, for good progress has been made.' I wish that my parents had taken that last comment to heart. I received a minus for creative writing, commenting that my spelling was a problem but I had good ideas. I received a satisfactory for maths and she also commented on my keen interest in science. But best of all, I received a plus for creative activities, where the teacher commented 'All art and craft work excellent. Very promising for the future. Music also good'. I hoped this meant that when I left school I could do a practical job, obviously there was some hope for me yet. Her overall comments were 'I am very pleased with Alison's progress this year. She has developed an interesting personality with many qualities. Yes - there will be some very hard work ahead - but I know she will persevere. My good wishes go with her.' The teacher's words 'very hard work ahead' and 'she will persevere' were to become more of a reality than any of us could have realised at this time. The sense of self-worth that she had helped grow within me was the greatest gift anyone could have given me at that time.

THREE

Separations

1

....September 1981. First Year Secondary School (I was aged 12 for most of this academic year)....I am thrown into a world where there is no tolerance of difference. It was to be another 6 years before anyone would realise that my problems reached beyond the boundaries of Dyslexia (e.g. reading, writing, reversal and memory difficulties). I was still completely oblivious to the fact that I perceived in a different way and therefore had no frame of reference by which to verbalise the differences.

My mum is shouting at me yet again,
    "Get a move on. Hurry up. Have you got everything ready?"
    "Yes", I nervously replied while coming down stairs, "Mum, please will you walk with me to school?" This is terrifying because I do not know the way. How will I ever find my way through the jungle of manic sensations all competing for my attention; smells, sounds of people, sounds of roaring cars, sounds of birds, all the visual chaotic movement, brightness, blurs of colour and bits of things which make no visual sense.
    "Now come on, you are old enough to make your own way to school. It is only a 7 minute walk.", answered my mother. I must try to justify my fear,
    "Mum, I don't know the way."
    "Honestly, what do you mean. We have been through this several times. Walk to the High Street. Walk down that little narrow road, turn left, then take the first right and as you walk down that road the school is on your right. We have lived in this village for 10 years and you should be able to find your way around by now. Anyway we have often driven and walked to near where the school is. How can you possibly not know the way?", said my mother in an irritated voice. Her instructions make no sense to me. The truth is I really do not know the way, I must convince my mother to show me the way,
    "Mum, I really don't know the way. Please will you walk there with me."
    "Alison, I am quite sure that the other children won't be walking to school with their mothers, since you are all now old enough to walk there on your own.", replied my mother as she began to become quite cross. I must persuade my mother somehow, so I will plead again,
    "I do not care whether the other children are walking on their own. The truth is I've no idea how to get to the school".
    "Okay, I'll walk with you. But you are to walk home on your own.", said my

mother despairingly.

"Please, could you come and collect me", I said hopefully.

"NO, no, I'll most certainly not.", replied my mother crossly. Oh well, it was worth a try! We walked outside down the drive way to the road.

"No, let go, you are not going to hold my hand. You are too old to hold my hand as we walk along. Your friends do not want to hold their mother's hand because it looks silly. You are old enough to behave in a more mature manner". I feel rejected by my mother. I find it very hard to walk outside without directly using someone as a reference, i.e. holding a person's hand. If there is no helping hand available I do not know where I am or where anything is in relation to me, resulting in disorientation and apparent clumsiness. If my actions are not considered 'normal' I get laughed at and pushed around by family and friends alike. I try so hard to behave normally. Why am I always failing?

As I walk down towards the school I feel nothing. All my emotions have been quashed; my mind is dominated by pure logical thought. The school seems like a huge maze, the multicolour blurs are running around manically, screaming and shouting. My inner strength of logical calm is a refuge from the external chaos. In amongst the pandemonium I stumble across one of the children from my previous school,

"Where are we supposed to be going?", I asked. She pointed vaguely towards a big door, and ran off. After a while we all ended up walking through that big door and sitting in a huge hall. I can only make out the odd word, which is being said by the teacher standing at the front of the hall. I feel so lost and alone. We are being spilt into groups and are being sent to a classroom. The only person known to me in my class is somebody from my previous school, who detests me. I choose to sit at the front of the classroom close to a wall. At least here the visual chaos is less.

After spending the whole of the morning in our Form Room we are sent to a French lesson. I just followed behind some of the people from my class. It is impossible for me to know or remember which way we went to get to the classroom for the French lesson. I am bewildered and disorientated. Again, to reduce the visual chaos I choose to sit at the front of the classroom by the wall. The teacher walks in and says,

"k(wl pqo4 f/;^&k alwe$i h~#kjy]ls". Is she talking English or French? I can barely hear or understand English when it is spoken, how will I ever manage French? As the lesson continues I am having terrible trouble understanding anything she says. I am never quite sure whether she is speaking English or French!

Next, we were sent to a mathematics lesson. At least here I can understand something of what the teacher is saying. In this school there are no stable references. For each lesson is in a different classroom. There is no desk, which is mine. The place is so large it appears to be an inconsistent labyrinth, and I just follow on behind any member from my class to get to our next classroom. I have no friends here and have been unable to understand the girl sitting next to me in the

Form Room. From the time I left home this morning I have been suffering from the paradox of being alone in a crowd. My logic is holding my fear and other emotions at bay. Why do most of the other people in my class seem to have some friends already? How can they understand what each other is saying? Why do the other children not seem as scared as I am? Why am I so incapable? I am good at quashing my emotional responses to these horrific situations. I no longer cry, thank goodness.

After what seemed like an eternity, it was time to leave. I ran the whole way home (fortunately I had remembered enough landmarks). But I did not want my mother to know how harrowing it was for me at secondary school because I knew she would be ashamed of me for being different from everybody else. So I told her that I'd had a good day!

From then on each day merged into the next. I loathe this school with its lack of security, caused by a shortage of stable references. The chaos seems never ending, my brain is permanently in overdrive, trying and failing to process all the different stimuli around me. We are expected to do so much work that my body always aches by the time I return home. Why does the school make us do homework when we are so tired? My mother has to help me do all my homework because I have little or no idea what anything is about. It is good that she is prepared to spend so much time helping me, but I just wish she would not become so frustrated with me and make me feel so useless. I cannot translate the words they use at school into anything meaningful. It is so demoralizing, my mother has terrible trouble explaining anything in a way that makes sense to me and also has immense difficulty understanding what I am trying to tell her. Why is it that on some days things are easier to do and on other days normally attainable things become unattainable?

After a few weeks I have made one friend. This is enough for the time being. She is my only tenuous link with security. At least I can now follow her to find my way around the chaotic labyrinth. It will be five years before I can leave this bedlam. How will I last out? This place is draining me.

Every day I aim to be the first out of the school gate. I run the whole way home. It is frightening trying to determine visual reality from illusion. Sometimes at the blurred peripheries of my vision I see shadows that at a glance appear to form a person's figure. At school where it is crowded, it is hard to know whether the shadows are real people or optical illusions. At school in a crowed corridor it is impossible to determine whether the shadows are real or apparitions. However, often when I am running home from school through the empty streets, I see what looks like a person walking or running behind me but when I turn around there's nobody there. This is very unnerving. How do other people manage not to become freaked by these optical illusions? Why am I so feeble?

It is embarrassing. While the rest of my form are all together doing English, I have to go to a remedial English lesson. The main advantage of being here is that it is quieter, with fewer people. I find all the remedial teachers very annoying because they do not appear to understand anything about Dyslexia and always seem to treat me as if I am unintelligent. I am told that Dyslexia is not recognised as a condition in its own right and that I have so called 'learning difficulties'. I find this infuriating because I consider Dyslexia to be the specific reason why I have 'learning difficulties'. I also believe that there are a variety of reasons why someone may have difficulty learning to read, write etc. and that each reason requires its own unique type of help. The work I do in remedial lessons appears to be geared towards people of low intelligence and not towards people with Dyslexia. I can do much of the work by simply using my intelligence, rather than any English skills. We are often asked to read a passage and then we answer questions on it. However, it seems that many of the passages relate to general knowledge subjects and I can often answer all the questions with the minimal amount of reading!

Surely the teacher has made a mistake. He has marked wrong, the question, which seems to be asking 'What controls the ocean tides?' I of course know that they are definitely the result of the moon's orbit around the earth. I have been told to reread the passage and find the correct answer to the question. I cannot imagine what the question means if the answer is not 'the moon', I have no doubt that the moon's gravity primarily controls the tides. After reading the passage the whole way through I went back to him and said,

"I know it is the moon which controls the tides, therefore my answer is correct", the teacher pointed towards a word in the passage.

"Wind", I exclaimed! "The wind definitely does not control the tides. I am not going to change my answer to wind!", I said firmly. It seems to me that they teach false information? If that is true, surely it is irresponsible! There appears to be an inconsistency. Either this teacher misunderstands the basics of physics or I misunderstand what is trying to be taught?

Science lessons are as much a disaster as English. We do these meaningless experiments. We must observe what happens and record our results. This is all very well except it is never explained why things happen. I can only remember why things happen and am completely useless at remembering a list of facts with no apparent connections or meaning. I am still unsure whether the French teacher is speaking English or French. Each time I go to the French class I sit there wishing that I could melt into the background, so that I will not be asked to read either some French or English. I dislike displaying my severe lack of ability because the other children find it funny. I hate giving the other children further ammunition to mock me.

Often I find the words the teachers use hilarious. It can be very amusing to hear only a few words from a sentence. In addition many people move their arms around in a peculiar way and pull strange facial expressions while they are talking. As a consequence of the odd words and actions the teachers make, I laugh. But strangely, the other children do not know what I find so amusing. At primary school, nobody minded when I laughed at the teachers, the other pupils just accepted it. However, here at secondary school everyone mocks me, because during the lessons I am always laughing alone. But in lessons when the other pupils are laughing I do not normally know what is humorous. Since it is my ambition to try and be 'normal' I am going to have to quash my sense of humour and try not to laugh unless the rest of the class is laughing. I just cannot be bothered with all this continual bitchy stuff, it seems so pointless, a waste of valuable energy. I rarely defend myself, but rather try and keep out of the way of trouble. Paradoxically, the best defence is silence, they get bored when I do not take the bait and if I am surrounded by a mob of people, I have discovered the best way to avoid getting beaten up is to silently walk away. My enemies do not know how to fight my silence.

In art lessons, we are asked to shade our drawings with light and dark areas. This seems completely daft because no object has a stationary shadow across it. Basically I am useless at everything we are asked to do; it does not matter whether it is Art, PE, Geography, Mathematics etc. I have terrible trouble understanding anything anybody says, or writes on the blackboard. I am making very little consistent sense of any of the work, everything seems equally irrelevant and a long way off from where I am.

Even in mathematics I have been put into the bottom group. Usually my reading is not good enough to be able to read the questions and so obtaining the correct answer is nearly impossible. Even if I manage to read the words in the question they often do not mean anything to me.

"Today we are going to study the number line.", shouted the teacher over the sea of deafening voices. As I look down at the page and gaze at the number line it completely dumbfounds me:-

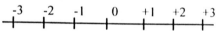

The teacher explains we can count below zero with minus numbers. I did not need to hear any more. This is not a twisted number system, it is straight (i.e. linear) just the way I always imagined it should be. I was right. I am absolutely livid with my father; he must be an absolute fool. It is possible to subtract a large number from a small number. I just want to continually shout, 'I have known that since the beginning of junior school but everybody told me I was wrong', but I will refrain. That evening I said,

"Dad it is possible to subtract either way, we did it in class today, look!".

"I know", he replied casually. He must really think that I am so stupid that I could not even work out something so obvious for myself. I have no way of expressing my frustration, I am so angry with my father. He is always saying to 'Tick-tock' Nana,

"I do not know how I managed to produce two children who are both so completely useless at mathematics". If only he had listened to me he would know that I am not totally ignorant. My father is always making me out to be worse than

I really am. He is often telling 'Tick-tock' Nana that my bedroom is very messy. My father does not know what he is talking about. Everything in my room is laid out so that I can find it and is kept in a constant, orderly, logical place. Surely, since everything is kept in a logical place my bedroom must be tidy. If an object is moved slightly I may trip over it or if someone puts an object in the wrong place (e.g. on my bed instead of my desk) it takes ages to scan my eyes across the whole room to find it. So what if many of the things are always laid out on my floor and desk. The room does not look messy to me. Fortunately, 'Tick-tock' Nana never takes any notice and still believes in me and considers me to be intelligent. She is my favourite person in the whole world, because she has faith in me and considers me to be worth something.

Perhaps I can find a way of making my father realise that I am not a complete failure. He seems to like people with something he calls 'character'. The people who my father considers to have 'character' are always making the people around them laugh. This means that I must find out how to make people laugh and then I will have 'character'. Then perhaps my father will like me more. I will observe what makes people laugh. It is hard to find the consistency and patterns in humour because everyone seems to find different things funny. Maybe one day I will understand enough about humour to make people laugh. Is there an overall solution to the subject of 'humour'?

I can solve practical problems that make sense to me. After a few months of trying to solve Rubik's Cube I finally succeeded (just before my 12th birthday). Put the pieces in any position and I can put it right within about 5 minutes, using the methods that I have derived without any help from anyone. (I never had access to, or the ability to read any of the solution books nor did I know anyone who could solve it.) My method is not the quickest, but why does nobody seem to notice that this must prove I am not a dimwit? (To this day, I have not met anyone else who has, without any help, worked out a method for consistently solving Rubik's Cube! I guess there are not that many of us!) My parents cannot solve this puzzle, so how can they still treat me as if I am so daft?

Jenny and I were outside playing on our bikes.

"I am going to run away. I hate living here. I do not feel as if I belong in this family. I am not joking. I really mean it", I explained to Jenny,

"Those people called mum and dad hate me. I am probably adopted. It is the only way I can explain the harsh way they treat me. I shall escape through the front bedroom window after we have been put to bed." (Jenny told me, years later, that she was really worried and did not know how to help me, but she did not want to be left behind with our parents while they were in such a bad mood!). However, with my lack of security I never did run away. I might have despised living at home, but I was too scared of the chaotic environment to even go to the shops on errands for my mother, partly because I had no idea of how to interact with the shop assistants.

I have trouble communicating with most of the people in my class; many of them seem to hate me. Why, I do not know. I dread the situation in lessons when we are told to get into groups; nobody ever wants me. I know that I am a social outcast. Generally I try and stay out of everyone's way, so there could be nothing worse than going away on a school trip with them all. I trust nobody at the school and I am unable to use anybody as a firm reference point. I spoke to my mother,

"Mum, I really do not want to go away on the school trip."

"For goodness sake. Not this conversation again. You are going. You will have fun. It'll be good for you. It's a wonderful opportunity to go to France for a week with the school", replied my mother. She does not understand. There is no way that I am going. I have been unable to make my mother back down, so I will have to be too ill to go away,

"Mum, my throat is very sore", I said.

"Well I am taking you to the doctors. You must be well enough for your trip to France next week", replied my mother. There is no way that I will let myself recover before next week. The sore throat continued and my mother was still talking about my trip to France. I became so frightened that I could not bear to be left on my own and my parents had to take turns sitting with me at my bedside. (My parents thought I was having a funny turn because I was ill and did not realise, until many years later, what was actually going on.) My mother came into my room and said,

"Tomorrow you are due to go to France".

"I don't feel well enough to go", I replied. Surely after being ill the whole week she would not make me go to France.

"I'm sure you will feel better by tomorrow", answered my mother. Her voice cuts through me like ice. There is nothing, which will make me go to France, with children who despise me and where there are no stable references. The thought of travelling on a boat across the English Channel has been giving me nightmares for weeks. At least when I go on holiday with my family they are my references and when I went camping last year with the school the headmistress was my reference. My mother continued,

"I am going to pack your suitcase for you". How could she do this to me? Why does she not understand? Is she heartless? My mother packed my suitcase but my will power was stronger than hers was and when it came to the next morning I refused to get out of bed saying that I was still too ill. It was a close shave! My classmates must be much more confident than me and much better at controlling their fears. Why am I such a weak person?

As the year progressed, many of my classmates became aware that I was in the remedial English class. Anyone who was in a remedial class was a potential object of ridicule. Each teacher that taught me was supposed to have been informed of my reading and writing problems, but cruelly it seemed to me as if this information never reached my teachers. I had endless problems. I would often be publicly reprimanded for carelessness in my written work and even worse, occasionally the teachers would ask me to read aloud to the whole class, which was funny for everybody, except me! The whole situation was brought to the fore one morning in July when the whole of my year was gathered during a morning assembly. It was a prize giving day. After a long while the person leading the ceremony began talking about the remedial English class awards and as far as I could understand he claimed that those in the remedial class were at 'the other end of the scale'. This seemed to me to be an incredibly patronising comment. My remedial English project won an award, it was supposed to be a profile about myself, but I ended up discussing the mysteries of quasars and the possibility of errors in the red shift! I went up onto the platform and received the award, some book tokens, an ironic prize for someone who had no interest in reading! After this, nearly everybody in the whole year considered me to be thick. Often the people in remedial classes were considered to be 'un-cool to be friendly with' and were very often given a rough time by many of the other pupils and some teachers.

    My parents decided that they should have an Educational Psychologist come and assess me on a private basis. Unbeknown to me, they wanted to know if I was intelligent, or whether they were just kidding themselves in thinking that my intellect was fine. Also, unbeknown to me, they decided that if I were intelligent they would personally help and put pressure on me to achieve my potential. The tests revealed that in some areas I was very bright (e.g. shapes) and in others I was very backward (e.g. mental arithmetic, short-term/working memory), but on average I had an IQ of about 110, which is considered to be 'at least average intelligence'. (In hindsight, it is obvious that some of the tests would have been a measure of my disability rather than my ability, since the tests take no account of poor vision etc.) The extremely uneven profile of abilities suggested Dyslexia, but despite this I still slipped through the holes in the education net and remained struggling on my own, without the help I needed.

    By the end of the year I knew a few more people. Despite putting everything into my academic work I did very badly in the end of year exams. Although I wanted to be 'normal' and able to learn, nothing ever penetrated my language barrier. Most things we were taught seemed to lack relevance and consistency, so they made no sense to me. My inability to read was also a tremendous handicap. I passed mathematics and music but I disastrously failed every other subject. My marks were so low that in each subject I was always very near or at the bottom of my class. The only subjects we had been streamed in during the first year were mathematics and French. I was in the bottom stream for both. I achieved the second highest mark in my mathematics class but was not allowed to move up to the middle stream because I could not read! In addition, I failed to attain the certificate in basic French, which the vast majority of the other children had achieved. My French vocabulary literally only contained a few spoken words, I could not consistently spell, pronounce or read any other French word. I had made some progress in my English, driven by a deep desire to go back into the main stream English lessons, but my reading age was equivalent to that of a slow and hesitant 8-year-old.

2

....Second Year Secondary School (I was aged 13 for most of this academic year).... I was placed in the bottom stream for all subjects and I appeared to be one of the most incapable students in my school year.

I have hardened myself to the terror of this school. I try to use logic as opposed to emotion. To help me make some sense of the chaos, in each different classroom we attend, I always choose a desk which is at the front of the room, preferably near a wall. There are less visual distractions by a wall. Any reduction in visual chaos that I can achieve is very worth while. From the front of the classroom I can see the blackboard and hear the teacher more easily. The remedial department is the exception. Small groups of desks are set up between partitions. This is bad because the partitions are not soundproof which means the voice from the person teaching my group becomes intertwined with all the other voices from behind the other partitions.

At last, it's happened. I have been given the option of returning to the mainstream English group. What a relief. Now at last, maybe some of my classmates will treat me as if I am human. Hopefully some of the mockery will cease. The strange thing is, I can not read anywhere near as well as my friends and my spelling is very poor. Why am I allowed to return to the mainstream group when my English is still about four years behind my chronological age?!

Occasionally the teachers will ask members of the class to read out aloud to the whole class. In all the lessons my worst fear is that I will be asked. Since my reading is so poor, many of the other pupils in the class snigger as I make an endless round of mistakes and hesitations. However, the taunting has motivated me to try even harder to learn to read. I have even been doing a modest amount of reading at home. If I read continually for more than a quarter of an hour I become totally exhausted, so I try to limit my time spent reading. Despite all my efforts, my reading age is still only that of a very slow, hesitant 9 year old.

I search endlessly to try to make some consistent sense of the English language, both spoken and written. Often, during a period of days or weeks, I repeatedly ask my parents a question. In their answers my parents use completely different words to describe the same thing. Sometimes they appear to give completely different answers. I need to keep asking the questions so that one day I can find some sort of continuity in the English Language and consistency about my surroundings. The older I become the more angry and irritated they become, when I repeat questions. If only there was a way for me to explain what I am doing. My parents often help me with my homework because I have not normally understood the day's work at school. They become very frustrated. They have to keep explaining things until they find a way that I can understand. Just changing a few words or their order can make the difference between total comprehension or complete misunderstanding. If the concept is new I need to be able to understand it as a whole, before any of the details make consistent sense. It is useless trying to expect me to remember a few apparently unrelated facts, because I need to instantly understand their interconnection to build a memorable concept in my mind. Although, often what people explain is not a new concept to me, it is just that the words make no sense.

Even my handwriting is wrong. My parents are always saying, 'You should learn to hold a pen properly and not wrap your thumb around the top of your index finger. It is not surprising that you write so slowly when you hold the pen so extremely tightly and awkwardly. Why do you have to press so hard? You indent a few pages under the one that you are writing on. Why do you have to write such large letters? Your style is so immature'. I have tried without success, to follow their advice about holding the pen, writing smaller and not digging my pen into the page. If I did not hold the pen tightly, I am sure my hand, arm and shoulder would not become so tired and painful. It is just so hard to write, that I have to do it my way otherwise the pen is uncontrollable and my writing illegible.

I cannot even hold a dessert spoon 'properly' my parents say 'You are old enough to use a spoon properly. A spoon is not a shovel'. However, if I try to hold the spoon 'properly' I then get into trouble for spilling my food! I get fed up with being continually told about all the things that I do wrongly. It often feels as if I never do anything correctly.

At last we are going to study Physics. This is something that I have always wanted to do. Unfortunately there is one snag. As usual, I can hear very little of what the teacher says and this is severely hindering my progress. I wonder how the other pupils in my class have overcome this problem? The most logical solution seems to me, to learn to lip-read. Although this is not easy because it is hard to keep my eyes focused on moving objects e.g. someone's lips. Over a period of several months, at every opportunity, I have tried to teach myself to lip-read. I am becoming good enough to fill in most of the gaps in my hearing. Combining the visual information from lip-reading and the sound of a person's voice, I can now work out most of the spoken words. However, actually interpreting the words into something meaningful is a totally different matter.

This new lip-reading tool has opened up a whole new world. Now, I can pick out many of the words spoken by the physics teacher, the other teachers and fellow pupils. I do not boast about my new lip-reading skills. I am sure that everybody else must have been lip-reading for many years before I realised it to be the solution to grasping speech. Maybe my new found lip-reading skills will enable me to learn to better distinguish between sounds I hear and so reduce my dread of the telephone. Perhaps it is necessary to lip-read in order to learn to hear all the subtle sounds of the English language. Why has it taken me until now to realise the need for lip-reading? Why am I so far behind my peer group in realising how to cope with, and behave normally? I must be so slow.

There are so many things that I do not understand. For instance, it is obviously as easy to read text in the correct orientation as it is to read text in any other orientation (e.g. upside down), letters look the same whichever angle they are viewed. During informal exams, to ensure we are unable to copy answers from each other, we are often made to sit at opposite sides of the desks facing each other (rather than next to each other). Why do the teachers not realise that we can read upside down writing? Putting us opposite each other actually makes it very easy to discreetly copy answers, or get ideas from another's work!

I am bored in the bottom stream of mathematics. I have worked through the textbook far beyond the place of the rest of the class. Rather than understanding the principles of the mathematics, I use my self-devised, abstract logic pattern matching theories, to obtain the correct answers. Most of the principles of mathematics are beyond me, because the language used to describe them does not make any sense. It has been decided that because I am so far ahead of the rest of my group and those in the middle stream, that I should study from the same textbook as those in the top stream, who are studying matrixes. I have repeatedly asked to be moved out of the bottom stream, but receive the same reply each time, 'there is no room for you in the middle stream'. It is completely unjust and very frustrating. Since I am now doing the same work as the top stream surely they could put me there? Perhaps given the right opportunity I could be good at mathematics?

I am completely useless at PE (sports) I am always falling over and can do very little of what is required of me. When I was a child my mother sent me to ballet dancing lessons, but they did not do me any good! Most of the PE activities are far beyond my meagre capabilities. I cannot run fast, hit or catch a ball or even jump over the 'horse' in Gymnastics. I am just too slow. The one activity I can do is cross-country running and this is only because I can run through the pain barriers and just keep going. During a Cross Country race I experience increasingly terrible pain in my limbs, shoulders and chest, but each time I defeat the pain just so that I can be reasonable at something. As exhaustion consumes me during a race (or at any time when I am tired) it becomes more difficult for me to control my balance to prevent myself from falling over. Everything else I try in PE goes completely wrong. Often, when I do the wrong things, I get into trouble for not paying attention. I do pay attention, but I am so terrible at comprehending even the simplest of instructions that it appears that I am purposely misbehaving.

One of my friends has taken to slapping me around the face. She finds it very amusing that I never notice her hand accelerating towards my face, until it has made contact. Which means I am unable to brace myself, let alone make an evasive manoeuvre. My friend's behaviour irritates me because I can never get my own back, since she always sees my hand coming. I take this annoying trait of my friend in the fun spirit in which it is delivered, but this behaviour is not acceptable from my mother. The violent slaps around the face from my mother, make me feel nothing more than repulsion towards her. Surely, she can see that I am too slow to even brace myself. Often I do not realise what has happened until moments after the incident. It is usually her frustration with me for being so slow, which causes her to lash out. I feel only despair that I cannot verbalise my disgust.

My mother gets endlessly frustrated with me, I never do anything well enough. She tries to help me with such things as homework, but I find her anger intolerable. Often my parents call me an 'idiot' and this has made me feel even more worthless. I dread to think what they would call me if they realised the number of things that are beyond me and the extent of my inability to cope with pain. My mother calls herself a Christian. I do not want to have anything to do with Christians if this is typical of their behaviour, but perhaps she is a good person? In which case I am very bad, beyond redemption.

My parents try to open up opportunities for me. They, like myself, are eager for me to find a niche in life. I have been allowed to stop my piano lessons, since this is definitely not my forte! Instead I have started to learn to play the flute. Having only one stave to read makes this instrument much easier for me to learn and within 4 months of starting, I passed the grade 3 examination. At last I have succeeded in something! Not only that, I have received some good marks in some of my end of year exams. This improvement is mainly due to my new found skills in lip-reading and remembering the spoken word, rather than relying on my poor attempts at reading it. Often I do not understand the real meaning of the words but I can work out and remember enough to get by.

3

....Third Year Secondary School (I was aged 14 for most of this academic year).... With the academic help my parents had given me combined with much hard work from myself, I managed to climb from the bottom streams in History, Geography and Mathematics into the middle streams.

Each day I try to act as normal as possible. Every time I slip up there is someone waiting to tell me how unintelligent or abnormal I am. The continual mockery from all sectors motivates me to try ever harder to behave within the expectations and boundaries of conventional society. There are too many constraints and protocols. Everything about me is wrong, the way I speak, look, walk, behave, how will I ever manage to bridge the gaps. It is mind-boggling.

My mother is always telling me to stop kneeling on chairs and sit properly and also to walk in a 'lady like' fashion. I do not have the slightest idea what she is talking about. She says I should walk slower, take smaller strides and keep my legs much closer together. She must know that it is hard to stand up and walk along without falling over, obviously everyone needs to brace their muscles, particularly in the neck, back and legs. Besides, I am not aware of which aspect of my walking style is wrong or how to correct it and cannot see the difference between the way I walk and the way everybody else walks. A couple of years ago my mother decided that I was now old enough to walk down the street without holding her hand. I feel rejected. She has deprived me of my best frame of reference. Now when I walk down the street or through the shopping centre, I hold onto her shopping bag, so that I have some idea of where she is relative to myself. However, she does not take me into account and despite rapidly compensating and trying to judge where I am in relation to all the manic movement of the people, I still regularly bump into things. Shopping is exhausting. How do other people cope?

My father is always saying that I 'go around like a bull in a china shop', but I do my best to control my clumsiness. I hold my muscles tightly but I am just not good enough at controlling my body. Why does everybody put so much emphasis on things that I consider irrelevant? Surely it is more important what sort of person I am?

One of my worst problems occurs when playing badminton. Apart from having the normal problem of making my eyes see the shuttlecock, I seem to fall over much too often. The others in the class mock me. The worst time is when doing an overhead clear. I pull the racket back over my shoulder and look up high into the ceiling of the sports hall for the descending shuttlecock, but as soon as I look up into the ceiling I fall over backwards. I always fall straight backwards to the floor, cracking my head on the ground, long before I even realise that my body has fallen, therefore I can never use my hands to save myself! Even when I fall forwards, I do not always manage to realise in time to put my hands out to save myself. I am so stupid that I cannot even control my own balance like other people.

Worse still is when we are playing team sports. I cannot process the information in front of my eyes quickly enough to see who is wearing the same colour top as myself. In addition, I sometimes see the wrong colour. Often I will glance at a green object and I will see it as orange, or vice versa. This means that if we are playing Netball and someone is wearing a green top I may distinctly see it as orange. So when I have the Netball in my hands and everybody is rushing around me waiting for me to throw it, I have no idea who is on my team. I have a 50% chance of throwing it to someone on my team, before I am disqualified for holding the ball for too long. I tell the other children that I am colour blind. This is my only way of explaining the problem. I just never seem to see things as quickly as other people. Am I just slow? Or does my short-sightedness, which is corrected by glasses, still cause me problems.

Being volunteered by my peers to read out aloud in class is not isolated to any one lesson. My reading is so poor that I find it extremely traumatic and embarrassing to attempt it in front of a class full of 'normal' people. To make matters worse I often find that my articulation worsens considerably when I am tired or in stressful situations. There are many who find it very amusing when I read. In some of the classes, a particular friend whispers the words in my ear, so I do not make a complete hash of reading the passage out aloud. At least most teachers do not literally laugh at me.

Unfortunately, several times a week I encounter a particular teacher who often wishes certain passages to be read out aloud to the whole class. Every time this particular teacher asks for a volunteer to read, there is a persistent loud chorus of voices shouting my name. As far as I can understand they wish me to read because it disrupts the flow of the lesson and gives them something to laugh at. This particular teacher invariably gives in, resulting in me having to read the passage. The problem is I only have the reading age of a 10-year-old and most of the words in the passages are far beyond my level. As a result I stumble over a great many of the words. Often this particular teacher has to tell me what a word is. This particular teacher stands, leaning on her desk and along with the rest of the class, laughs at my attempts to read. Even those I would call my friends laugh at me. It is completely degrading and demoralising. I feel worse than useless. It does not matter how hard I try, I just seem unable to read. I would not normally tell my mother about the mockery I endure at school because it is obviously my fault for being such a dunce, but I am going to make an exception in the case of this particular teacher. I believe that even my mother would not approve of any teacher regularly laughing at my inability to read. I believe this particular teacher is behaving disgracefully. As we ate our diner I nervously started to broach the subject of this particular teacher by saying,

"Mum, 'X' isn't a very nice person."

"Alison, that is not true.", said Jenny, "I have that teacher. That teacher is a lovely, kind and caring person". I replied anxiously,

"That is not true...".

"That teacher is a wonderful person", interrupted Jenny.

I may as well give up now. If this particular teacher is all that Jenny says, I must deserve to be laughed at. Evidently it is my fault that this particular teacher abuses me. My mother would probably say that if I bothered to learn to read I would not have these social problems.

I have observed that one channel of normal social contact, which my peers engage in, seems to be the mutual enjoyment of pop music, but even this is beyond me. I cannot hear the words, or remember them, when my friends sing them to me. It perplexes me as to how they manage to catch the words and remember them. It is very annoying. To discover the words in a given song I have to listen to it very many times (e.g. 50 times). Even when I do find out what the words are, the poetic language seems incomprehensible. My patience does not stretch that far so I ignore pop music in preference to orchestral classical music. Among other things my classmates find my preference for classical music very peculiar! Why?

The older I become the more things I am expected to do and the more things I fail at. I have recently seen a programme on the television about an agoraphobic lady who has been trapped in her house for many years and is too scared to even walk to the end of the street. I can relate to the way this lady feels, but why? I am not agoraphobic. I do not faint or go all peculiar when I go outside. My house is never going to become my prison. Does my empathy mean I am a hypochondriac?

I have a headache after eating certain foods such as eggs or drinking milk, also a stomachache after drinking orange juice. How can this be? I must be imagining it. Reading gives me a headache. All sorts of things cause pains in my body. Nobody believes that reading gives me a headache so how could they believe the rest. Is the pain real or imagined? Perhaps I am mentally infirm. I had better not let anyone notice my mental inadequacies in case I am sent to the psychologist or psychiatrist. Being at school must be better than being locked away in an institution for people who are mentally ill.

At school we are all required to choose which subjects to pursue in the next two years. Unfortunately it is the school's policy that we all study a foreign language. I have been unable to make any consistent sense of the French language because I cannot hear and pick out the sounds. After studying it for 3 years, my vocabulary is literally limited to about 7 words, none of which I can spell or read! My French is so bad that there is no one in my year worse than I am. We have all been studying German for the past 2 years and since the phonetics, sounds and spellings are similar to those in the English language, this has enabled me to make some limited progress. Therefore continuing with German is my only option. We must all study English language, English literature, Mathematics and European studies. In addition I have chosen to do Technical Drawing, Physics, Geography and Music. Having already achieved grade 5 in the Theory of Music and studying for grade 5 in Flute, the music course should be within my grasp.

I would have continued doing Art but my work is not good enough. I seem unable to understand the usual convention for shading drawings. Apparently my work lacks something called 'flow', my drawings contain too many stark straight lines rather than flowing together in a continuous fashion. Strangely, the teacher always insists I should draw an object from the angle that I am viewing it, rather than the angle which I prefer. Why should we draw an object from the angle at which we are viewing it, when it is so simple to draw it from any other angle? This year I have been doing woodwork and despite extreme physical pain and effort have proudly produced a good coffee table. At last I have achieved something tangible. (Now, in 1997, my table is still standing strong, despite having been regularly sat on! It sits in our living room).

I seem to be much slower at catching onto things than other people. I wish I could be good at just one thing. I do not care what it is. Surely there must be something that I can do, or am I just incapable of doing anything. I have always been determined that when I grow up I will not be nasty or abusive to anyone and definitely not to people who are different. I am committed to giving everybody a fair go and perhaps in the future I will be able to help people like myself.

FOUR

Marooned In Desolation

1

....*September 1984 Fourth and fifth Year Secondary School (I was aged 15 to 16 for these academic years)....I was under enormous pressure from all sectors to prove that despite my Dyslexia I had ability and tenacity to pass some GCE exams (equivalent to GCSE's) By this time I was in the top stream for Geography and the middle streams for Physics, Mathematics, English, European Studies and in the bottom stream for German. In the school that I attended, those who were in the middle stream or above were aiming to achieve at least a grade C at GCE (equivalent to a GCSE 'grade C'). My parents continue to help as best as they can and my hard work will hopefully pay off. There is no short cut to overcoming Dyslexia.*

Each day blends into the next. It is a continual circle of ridicule and severe pain. I wake up each morning hoping like crazy, that today, things will start to get better and I will be in less pain than the night before.

Every day I am acutely aware that I must do my best, to give myself any chance of obtaining the required marks in the forthcoming GCE. My parents say unless I achieve grades of C or better, my qualifications will be worthless. I try desperately hard to behave in a way which is acceptable to 'the world'. Knowing how to conduct myself in an acceptable manner is a lifetime's quest.

At school my classmates hassle me for not dressing in a trendy way or because I am not as quick as they are. I do not care about anyone else's appearances so why should I care about my own? For instance, does it really matter if someone does not have the latest fashion in uncomfortable shoes? Why wear materials/ clothes that are tight or rough? Why would I want to wear tights when they strangle my legs and make me feel as if billions of ants are running manically all over my legs? Why would anyone put up with such sensations? My classmates view the world in such a different way from myself, that there is really very little that we have in common. I have a few friends but they do not understand my way of thinking. Mostly I behave in the way they expect me to rather than in my natural way. For example, when someone tells a joke I just laugh at the same time as everybody else. It is not a true heartfelt laugh. To me the jokes are not funny, even if I manage to work out the double entendre. I simply try to conform and behave in the expected way.

I attempt to make sense of the work we do. It is so hard to interface between 'my world' and 'the world'. It is often so hard to translate all the words into my own abstract thought patterns. As I read from the blackboards and the pages of the textbooks, my eyes become excruciatingly painful and all visual chaos makes me feel dizzy. When I try to plot graphs onto graph paper, it is very difficult to put the plot in the correct position, because as I endeavour to follow the lines up and across the paper, they keep disappearing. Equally as I strive to follow the contour lines on a map, they also disappear, even if I follow them with my finger. My arms and shoulders continuously ache from all the writing and my whole body becomes physically tired. Everyday I struggle through several pain barriers, often using a mental strategy to send parts of my body partially numb. I literally think the pain away. It is the only way I can survive such constant pain.

After a harrowing, painful, tiring day at school, I return home to the pressures, expectations, and frustrations of my parents. I am unsure which is worse, being at home or at school. My parents believe that by pressuring me it will motivate me to fulfil my potential, but the pressure is destroying me. My father often says 'I know you better than you know yourself'. If this is true why do my parents treat me so harshly? I am not at all sure that I can live up to their expectations. My parents expect me to behave and act normally in the world, then become frustrated and cross with me when I fail. Often, when I refuse to practise my reading, my father says things such as 'you are your own worst enemy'. I am too weak to completely overcome the pain and as exhaustion sets in my eyesight deteriorates. Sometimes, I cannot simultaneously see one whole letter on a page of average sized print. Imagine the effort required in attempting to read a word, while only seeing a part of a single letter at any given time. How do other people cope with these visual distortions?

My mother has told me that when people read quickly, 'they may just read a few words from each line while moving their eyes straight down the centre of the page' (as opposed to moving their eyes along the line and reading each word, or in my case, letter). I have tried this but it does not seem to work for me. Several times I have read a few words from the approximate centre of each line of a passage, but it never makes any sense. Apart from anything else it is often quite hard to judge which are the middle words! I am amazed that normally people can understand a passage by reading so few words. My ability for the English language must be incredibly inferior and hopeless. How will I ever bridge such an immense gulf?

Each evening I study, trying to break through the pain, trying to do that thing called concentration. Concentration is an unattainable goal. How do other people manage it? Despite every effort my mind is continually and uncontrollably attracted to all stimuli. I cannot filter anything out, which means that everything becomes intertwined in my mind and I cannot sustain my attention on any task. Often my brain becomes overloaded causing me to become phased-out. Ideally I need a peaceful environment.

On top of all these problems there is one more, the sound from Jenny's radio. She does not have it blaring but my room is next to hers and the sound easily penetrates the thin walls. She listens to the radio as she does her homework and while she potters around in her room. The sound that my ears receive from her radio interferes with my thinking processes. The material that I am studying becomes intertwined with all the sounds from the radio and any other prominent stimuli (e.g. cooking smells, sound of footsteps/cars). This means my studying becomes that much harder to decipher and isolate from all the muddle of incoming distractions. This total inability to concentrate caused by things going on around me cannot be helped at school, but surely at home things could be different. I have asked Jenny to turn down the volume of the radio but she refuses and my parent's side with her. I have offered to buy Jenny a pair of headphones, but she has turned down my offer saying that she would not be able to use them because she moves around too much! My permanent exhaustion causes me to have no tolerance of my parents or Jenny's awkward behaviour and often in total frustration, instead of hitting out, which I now know to be socially unacceptable in 'the world', I slam my hand against a wall or doorpost. It is often hours later before I feel the pain and the bruises appear. If anyone ever asks how I cut and bruised my hands I always find some vague excuse.

Often, my homework takes me from the time I come home from school, until gone eight o'clock, by which time the exhaustion and pain have become too much to bare. There is not enough time in each evening to do all the homework, so the less urgent parts are left to the weekend. Normally once my homework is finished I just watch the television. During this time nobody hassles me. I need to be in bed by half past nine each night. I cannot physically keep my eyes open any later. Day after day of exhaustion is very draining, physically and emotionally.

I climb into bed each night like a zombie, devoid of all emotion and energy. To calm the chaos in my mind, I imagine that I am in a featureless desert and all I can see is the yellow sand stretching out in front of me, before finally meeting the blue cloudless sky. In my desert there are no people, sounds, sensations, smells or stimuli of any kind, just stillness and peace. This is the environment in which I would like to live. In the depths of my imagination I have made ghosts of people who are kind, loving and understanding. These ghosts of my mind exist to take the place of my normal turbulent human relationships. Maybe one day I will find such people. I fall asleep in the stillness of my mind, but without fail I am rudely awakened a few hours later with nightmares. I awake in a state of very high anxiety. My emotions and fears hunt me all day long, like hungry wild beasts, but while I am awake I can control and hide from them, but as soon as I sleep they rear their ugly heads. Once awake, it often takes me up to half an hour to calm down enough to return to my bed. This is my own private hell, I am too ashamed of my weakness to tell anyone of my disturbed sleep. I suffer in silence. Somehow I must find a way of further controlling my mind.

My weekends are no better than my weekdays. We are supposed to have about 2 or 3 hours homework each night, but often it takes me considerably longer. Consequently, the whole of Saturday and also Sunday morning is consumed with homework. On top of this my parents expect me to do simple tasks, like laying the table at meal times and drying the dishes after dinner. I have to put so much extra effort into doing many things that I quickly become fatigued and my lack of activity is often seen as laziness. To conserve energy, I tend to discern between what I consider to be essentials and nonessentials. When I fail to do tasks, my parents, sister and teachers accuse me of being lazy and often say, "Alison can do 'it' if she really wants to". Why do they insist I do these extra activities when I am obviously completely drained from trying to meet their academic expectations? Now that I am so busy with my homework, I seldom have the opportunity to visit the only person I respect in the whole world, 'Tick-tock' Nana. This is a huge blow. I miss her.

There are a few tiny glimmers of hope in this hell which most people call life. I have a private English teacher who comes to the house and she has been able to help me improve my written work and give me guidelines on how to answer exam questions. She is one of the very few people who does not grind me down. Additionally, every other Sunday night I go to a small Youth Group where we sit around having organised discussions and the occasional game. Often I have no idea what they are discussing because their words seem meaningless. The teenagers in this group never mock me, although I wait on tenterhooks for the day that changes. To be accepted for who I am just seems too good to be true!

It is said that 'no man is an island'. For me this statement is not true. In many respects I am now completely isolated. I cannot relate to anybody and nobody can relate to me. For the purposes of self-preservation I have separated my emotional self from the outside world. Not even one living entity on this earth really understands me. If there is a God in the universe does it understand me?

My Grandfather often says,

"School days are the best years of your life". If this were true I am not interested in living, there would be no point. My life has always been a huge solitary struggle. From the day I was born nobody has ever understood me, I have always been alone, perplexed, lost. Either I am very weak or very different from everybody else. I have no way of knowing how to cope with this total isolation and no way of communicating my predicament. The older I become the worse my life becomes, because I cannot interface between my world and the world. What is the point of living this life of mine, it is too hard.

I ask myself this question each day, why should I bother to live? Would it not be better to simply end my misery now? Surely there can be no point to my useless and hopeless life? I seem unable to make any proper contribution to society and find it hard to imagine that I ever will. Perhaps the creator of the universe had a warped sense of humour. At school I have heard the phrase 'To be or not to be', I have no idea where it comes from or who first said/wrote it but to me it is a summation of my struggle of whether to commit suicide or not. I do not feel that I can continue on like this indefinitely and if indeed school days are the best days of a person's life I do not wish to be around to discover what worse things life will throw at me.

At school, as part of our English lessons, we have discussed in some detail, the subject of suicide from the perspective of all parties involved. Having thought about what the teacher and others have said, I am not sure that my parents or particularly 'Tick-tock' Nana would cope if I committed suicide, so for their sake I will hold on a little longer just to see if things do become any better. I have told nobody of my intention to commit suicide, because after I have killed myself, I do not wish anyone to feel guilty for not trying harder to stop me. Sometimes in total desperation I pray 'please God, if you really exist and if you really care about me, end my misery and kill me off in an accident'. If things stay too bad for much longer, or if they get worse, I will without doubt end my life, probably by electrocution (clean, quick and easy if you know how!).

2

....During the mock GCE[4] and CSE[5] exams I achieved:-

66% in GCE Technical Drawing	65% in CSE European Studies
57% in " Physics	62% in " Mathematics
56% in " English Language	43% in " German
50% in " Geography	
42% in " Mathematics	
41% in " English Literature	
18% in " Music	

At the end of the fifth and final academic year of my secondary school life the final exams are looming. Despite putting every last bit of energy I have into my studying, my teachers seem to be unsure whether I will manage to attain GCE grade C (mark of greater than 50%) in most of the subjects in the actual exams....

There is one thing that I have always wanted to try and that is skiing! The school is organising a skiing trip for all those in the fifth year and I have decided to go. As we drive from the school in the coach I brace myself for the inevitable disorientation of travelling. None of my friends are on this trip and many of the people on this coach often taunt me. My only references are my bags, my seat and myself.

At Dover the coach boards the Ferry and we all leave the coach for the duration of the short sea journey across the English Channel. We all somehow end up in one of the lounges on the boat. I have no idea where the coach is in relation to this lounge. To prevent myself from becoming disorientated and dizzy I walk a few metres out onto the deck and watch the horizon for the duration of the crossing,

---

[4] between approximately 50% to 65% was needed to achieve a grade C

[5] A mark of between approximately 70% to 80% was required at CSE for an equivalent GCE grade C pass

periodically walking back inside, just to check that some of the people from our school party are still in the lounge. As we approach the dock, I walk back inside and to my horror everybody has gone. I have no idea of how to find my way back to the coach. What should I do now?! I am lost. I will have to stay here and hope they come and look for me. It's okay; I can see some people from my school. So I will follow them back to the coach.

We have travelled all night and arrived in the Austrian village the following day. The exhaustion has as usual caused me to become even more uncoordinated and trying to eat some dinner without disgracing myself is very hard. Once dinner is over I will collapse into bed.

Each day we go skiing, once in the morning and once in the afternoon. For the first few days it has been very cloudy and using all my ingenuity, tenacity and sheer strength, I have managed to control my body enough to ski! But today, the blinding sun came out and we have now graduated from the beginner nursery slope to a much steeper slope. I cannot see adequately because of the blinding sun and have no references to tell how steeply the ground was falling away below me. This is truly disorientating. All I can do is to follow the speed and angle of approach of the other people in the group and hope that they know what they are doing. Mostly this seems to be working, however if they go wrong so do I. I have to stay close to the other people in the group because I could easily lose them in the blinding sun. We are staying in a very small village with only one main road, which suits me because it makes it fairly easy to navigate myself around. My bed in the shared room is my reference point and sanctuary from chaos.

A sea of faces confronts us as we drive back into the school. Our parents are all waiting for us. I cannot distinguish my father from the crowd. I find that on the whole the difference in each human face is very subtle. In order to recognise a person, I make a mental note of their main features (e.g. thin, fat, young, old) and any dominant facial features (e.g. long hair, big nose!). A person's watch is a good indicator of their identity. There are so many different types of watch and on the whole watches vary from person to person. In addition, such things as the person's individual smell/perfume and sound of their voice are all useful indicators of identity. Trying to recognise my father from the coach window is therefore very difficult. Having narrowed it down to about three possibilities, I clamber off the coach hoping that he will come to me!

I told my parents that I had a brilliant time, which is true in one respect, but there is always a great cost for me to pay whenever I do anything - pain, tiredness, disorientation, etc. This holiday was no different from any of the other holidays or days out I have been on. Why does enjoyment always have to come at such a high price?

3

Make or break time has come. I will spend from May until the middle of June taking my exams. Having come this far, I have decided to do the exams and will consider the question of suicide after the exams. For the first time in my school life, because of my Dyslexia, I will be given extra time in my exams, which will give me a better chance of writing down all that I know. Emotionally there is nothing left of me, all my emotions have been quashed, I exist like a computer using only pure logic. I claw my way through each day, living for that day only, determined not to look either to the past or the future. Every day I work under excruciating pain and until my eyes will no longer function. The pain is so much part of my life I simply take it for granted. Why am I so feeble compared with everybody else? 'Tick-tock' Nana has become critically ill and is lying alone in a semi-coma in hospital. My parents will not let me go and visit her and I do not have the energy to insist that I go. I cannot imagine a future without her. She is the main reason why I have not committed suicide. If she dies and my quality of life does not improve there will be no reason to continue living.

If I pass my exams I have an Electronic Apprenticeship waiting for me with a local firm. At least this should lead to some sort of practical job and if the headmistress at the junior school was correct and I am indeed good at practical things, hopefully I will do okay. But supposing 'school days really are the best days of a person's life'? Unbeknown to my parents, I heard them talking last week. Their basic doubt was to whether I would ever be able to succeed at anything without possessing the ability to read properly. I can read, but only slower than normal conversational speech. My actual reading age is now that of a 12 year old. When I go to work I will just have to find ways of hiding my lack of reading ability. What will I do if my exam marks are not good enough to start the apprenticeship? What will happen if I fail the apprenticeship? Will I be able to hide my Dyslexia? The thought of being a total failure really scares me.

On the 16th of June, after completing the last of the torturous exams, I walked out of the school gates for the final time. At last I have finished school. Just for a brief moment I loosen the grip on my emotions. As I smile to myself I know that the 11-year school battle is over. What a relief. Sometime later a friend said,

"You must be a bit sad about leaving school"

"No, I hated it there", I replied,

"Yes, but surely there must have been a hint of regret at leaving", answered the friend. She understands nothing of my plight, thank goodness. Yet another person who thinks they understand the way I operate!

After lying in Hospital for four months, 'Tick-tock' Nana's life finally slipped away in the early hours of the morning. I was staying away from home at Shirley Nana's house and awoke from my sleep with a jerk. I knew the second I came to that she had died. Nobody needed to tell me (My mum came around later in the morning and told Shirley Nana and myself). The only person I had any affinity with had deserted me, but why? I am alone now and through necessity have lost the ability to cry. I can neither accept nor deal with any negative emotions. One very strong reason for carrying on living has been that I did not want to desert 'Tick-tock' Nana. But now she is dead. Perhaps now would be a good time for me to end my life. No, that would not be logical. I really ought to wait for my exam results just to make sure that I have failed them. No, I did work hard so perhaps I could have passed? If I have failed the exams I will have no future or prospects and will definitely commit suicide, by Electrocution.

Looking at the envelope in front of me will not change the exam results concealed inside. So I rip it open. Frantically, I cast my eyes down the list. A wave of relief and excitement comes over me. I have achieved a grade 1 CSE in Mathematics, English and European Studies (grade 1 in CSE is equivalent to GCSE grade C). In addition I achieved a grade 2 in music and a grade 3 in German. It will be several weeks before the GCE results are published but providing I have achieved a Grade C in Physics I will have fulfilled the entry requirements to start an Electronics Apprenticeship this coming September. (Grade C at GCE is equivalent to GCSE grade C.)

While I wait for the remainder of the results, my father has decided that I should practise my reading, as well as build a garden gate. Building a sturdy wooden gate is a doddle compared with the reading! (The gate is still standing strong today!) He has given me a science fiction book. The only way I can stop my father from hassling me is to show willing and read the 'stupid' book. However, this will be physically painful and tiring. To make matters even worse, I can at best only read at normal speaking speed and often my brain just overloads and stops working. I have decided to read the book at every possible moment, which means reading from the time I wake up in the morning to the time I go to bed in the evening. This way I can get all the pain over at once, rather than spreading it over many weeks. It took me approximately one week to read the book and about 3 weeks for my energy level and eyesight to recover. During the week I was reading the book, I became ever more tired and my eyesight deteriorated. By the time I finished the book my eyesight was so bad that it was hard to distinguish any of the letters. Despite the difficulties, I managed to vaguely grasp the general story line. This is the first and hopefully the last book I will ever read all the way through. (To this day the only other book I have read is the one I wrote!)

What is it about Dyslexia that makes me so tired? I am ashamed of my weakness and so I hide the tiredness and pain. My parents say that I should never use Dyslexia as an excuse for not doing something and neither should I hold it up like a banner. They insist that I must endeavour to hide and overcome the Dyslexia, so that nobody realises the extent of my problems. The older I become the more ingenious my strategies need to be. How will I ever cope on the Electronics Apprenticeship?

The day finally came when I received my GCE results. Just for a moment I let the guard down on my emotions, so that I could feel the joy. I attained a grade C in Physics, Technical Drawing, Geography, English Language and remarkably, in English Literature. I had relied entirely on my friends and mother reading to me the set books on the English Literature course! I would never have achieved any of these results without the academic help from my friends and parents. But was the achievement of these results really worth all the pain? My parents put so much emotional pressure on me that it nearly destroyed me. Were a few grades and a piece of paper really worth all that suffering? Why are my parents not ecstatic that I have met their expectations? My father says 'he must not praise me in case I acquire a big head'. My qualifications are based on things that belong to 'the world' and not 'my world'. In my lonely world I understand so much, but my thoughts are so advanced that they can neither be expressed in words or pictures. Can advanced thoughts be expressed in words? I must search for a way of expressing myself.

FIVE

Finding A Way

1

....September 1986. First year of Electronic Apprenticeship and day release to college (I was aged 17 for this academic year)....Many had been surprised that I had worked my way up to a high enough level to start an Apprenticeship. I had learnt enough about how people normally conduct themselves, to be able to appear relatively normal myself. I could now read and write basic sentences well enough to get by. In the minds of the people who knew me the question remained, can Alison really make something of her life?

The time has come to enter the big wide world. Using a foundation of logic, I have plucked up enough courage to decide to wait exactly one year before reassessing the suicide issue. If it is true that my working life is much worse than my school life, I will end it all before my 18th Birthday. The logic in my brain has blocked out all fears, therefore I neither fear nor feel anything. The logic filter I have constructed over my emotions attempts to block all emotion and only allows out fun and laughter, but not too much, for that would be tiring. If I find something hysterically funny I must not laugh too much because the shuddering that runs through my body is overwhelming and the pain in my back and stomach is crushing.

My first challenge of this apprenticeship is to survive the first week, camping on a nearby island with all the other first year students and apprentices. As usual I create references for myself. A tent, a corner in the communal hall, specific routes around the site so that I do not lose my way. It is very hard operating in an apparently normal fashion, in this hostile environment. At least here nobody knows me and therefore there is a complete absence of abuse. It seems uncannily odd to be without the abuse, but I intend to do my best to keep things this way.

Throughout the week, we have been attending various lectures and doing practical activities. I have noticed that other people have a much higher energy level than myself, consequently I have to go to sleep much earlier. This is not usually a problem at home, but here at the campsite, trying to go to bed unnoticed is proving challenging, but not impossible! At home, by about 9pm I always start to become extremely tired and have tremendous trouble functioning on any level. By 10pm it is impossible for me to stay awake.

I promised myself that once my school days were over, this would be the end of my academic life. However, part of the conditions of this Electronics Apprenticeship is that we all attend a College of Further Education one day each week, to acquire a BTEC Ordinary National Certificate in Electronic Engineering.

It is hard at this college to make references because everything just seems to be one whirling mush of chaos. The speed at which they lecture is too fast for me to translate the material into something meaningful within my mind. All I can do is to copy the notes from the blackboard and then try to decipher them later. I am finding the contents of the course extremely difficult to keep up with. The one large problem is that the day is so long. We start at 9 am and do not finish until 9pm! But at least here they are willing to help Dyslexic people, by being more tolerant of faulty English and allowing extra time in all exams. The lecturers and my fellow students are not abusive towards me. This seems too good to be true. Will it last?

Travelling to and from work is very challenging. I dislike travelling in any vehicle. It is hard to judge distance effectively, which results in disorientation. If we become stuck in a traffic jam and the car keeps stopping and starting, then the jerking upsets my balance, resulting in even more disorientation, because static objects keep moving past when the car is stationary. Worse still are roundabouts. They also cause total confusion because everything just blurs past my eyes. At present my father is diverting his journey to work so that he can drop me off at my work place, but this is not going to be a long-term arrangement. It will be just until I become used to going to work! On the way home I have to brace myself against the disorientation of the 15 minute dreaded bus journey! Travelling in buses causes greater disorientation than in cars because it is harder to see where we are going. How do other people cope so well with the confusion of travelling?

At work things are tough, but my perseverance is paying off. I have produced between acceptable and good work in all the mechanical areas such as metal work, milling, lathing etc. However, when lathing I have terrific trouble turning the handles in the correct direction, which has resulted in several pieces of my work being ruined. It is intensely frustrating when I need to restart the work. I still have enormous difficulty measuring accurately with a ruler. Somehow I find it hard to know which way I am reading the measurement. For instance, I may confuse 6.4cm with 5.6cm. I find the 6cm on the ruler and then look in the wrong direction when trying to determine the decimal part.

The good quality of my mechanical work has been made possible because during my time at school, I studied both metal and woodwork and learnt to use the basic tools such as saws, drilling machines and files etc. Often I would do woodwork at home and my grandfather patiently taught me to use the tools properly. I do find doing such work tiring and painful, but the results are satisfying.

As part of the apprenticeship we also did technical drawing and computer courses, which were fairly easy. At last I have found something that I can do to a reasonable level and nobody at work perceives me as a hopeless failure, which is quite refreshing. I dread each Friday morning because this is when we must do a 5-10 minute spoken presentation to the other six people in our group. This is very difficult for me, since I cannot read my crib notes and speak at the same time. It is impossible for me to make eye contact with any of the audience, because if my eyes move away from my notes I hesitate as I attempt to find my place in amongst all the moving chaos on the page. The alternative solution would be to put one point on each of a set of cards, but then I would have to keep moving my hands, which also disrupts my speech. My presentations are not fluently spoken but nobody seems overly worried. I do not know how the others in my group cope with these problems so effortlessly.

As a group, led by an instructor, we are often given wads of typed notes to work our way through. This is a dangerous time for me, my inability to read could be exposed, since we all take turns in reading paragraphs out aloud. I always anticipate the next paragraph I will need to read and work out all the words, while the other paragraphs are being read. I am unable to read it perfectly and fluently but at least nobody notices my true incompetence. However, this means that following and comprehending the subject matter is very difficult because I am so busy trying to cope with my reading disability.

My father is relatively slow at reading and recently has been sent by the company he works for, on a course that is designed to help people read faster. He has returned with some very peculiar ideas. Unfortunately, but understandably, he wishes to impart his new found skills and techniques on me. He informs me that when people read they make their eyes skip in an arc shape from one word to the next, focusing on each word as they go! I have tried to explain that I am unable to see a whole word all at once but my father says 'you must learn to see more'. How does someone learn to simultaneously see more? My father tells me that with practise I will be able to recognise whole words without reading the individual letters and insists that I should start reading the daily newspaper. My mother says that it is only young children learning to read who might read the individual letters. She is adamant that I must stop the bad habit of reading each letter separately. My parents do not know what they are talking about. I know that I cannot simultaneously see whole words; is this a symptom of Dyslexia? Surely it cannot be overcome?

How can practising my reading improve my vision, when the act of reading for more than about ten minutes actually makes my vision worse?! I always successfully avoid practising reading since it is so painful. My parents insist that reading is the only way to improve and mature my English.

My poor awareness of how to properly refer to myself using the English Language is causing problems. To me there is little difference between 'You' and 'I'. However, most people use 'I' to refer purely to themselves (e.g. I went shopping) and 'You' to refer to someone other than themselves. At work and college I am often so disassociated from what I am doing that it seems quite natural to use 'you' when referring to myself. Other people at work and college find my use of 'You', 'I' etc. amusing and sometimes irritating. They often tease me. In my attempts to act in a normal way I am trying very hard to learn to use the correct words when referring to other people and/or myself.

My inability to readily comprehend the English language causes endless problems. Such words as 'it' and 'that' often catch me out. Somehow I fail to follow the sentences and lose the meaning of what is being conveyed. A stark practical example of this is; when I was a child my parents often used to say 'don't do that' and were always angered by my apparent insolence when I asked 'don't do what?'! Sometimes at work I am given verbal instructions and then expected to execute them. I have trouble turning so many words into something meaningful. Often I need to ask people to repeat instructions, or I recompose the instruction to check I have the intended meaning.

Another common problem occurs when one of the training instructors gives me a verbal message to give to someone elsewhere on the site. It is hard enough to find the person in the labyrinth of this huge manufacturing site, but remembering the name of the person I am supposed to find is virtually impossible. If I manage to navigate myself to the right person they always receive a garbled message! Why don't I write myself a note? It is not that I cannot remember a message but rather that I never comprehended it in the first place because I cannot remember a string of unrelated words. I always ask the sender of the message to repeat it at least once, but hearing something twice or even three times is often insufficient. To ask any more times would make me seem ridiculous. It is equivalent to someone speaking a foreign language and asking me to relay a message when I only know a few words of that language.

My memory is definitely defective. I remember doing things, but am unable to recall when they happened. Each evening after I return home from work I relay all the day's activities to my mother to help improve my memory recall. In a few months my recall has already marginally improved. My mother does not realise that repeating the days activities is for my benefit and not hers.

After the first three months of the apprenticeship, we have finished all the mechanical aspects of the course and it is time to start the Electronics. Initially we have to learn to solder and wire joints to a high standard. I am finding this extremely difficult. My fine muscle control over my hands is not good or versatile enough and using tools such as a pair of wire cutters, wire strippers, pliers or a soldering iron is virtually impossible. It is taking me a long time to programme my brain to a level where these objects behave themselves in my hands!

After several months of much effort I have acquired enough muscle control to produce good soldering joints, but the cost is severe muscle pain throughout my body. I need to hold the muscles in my arm firmly and brace my whole body to do any delicate task that requires a reasonable degree of dexterity. One false movement by any part of my body will often make my hands move, this has often caused the pen to mark the page or the soldering iron to burn my hand. Doing something delicate with any part of my body causes severe pain after a few moments and also a sort of 'itchy tingly' feeling inside the muscles. How do the others cope so easily with this pain and appear to master delicate tasks so effortlessly?

The cool unemotional logic of an engineering environment is an ideal place for me. I view all external things using only logic. Here, I am left to my own devices, which suits me fine. There is of course the usual banter but I am not vindictively hassled. Unfortunately, my lack of energy stops me from socialising at the pub at lunchtime or any time after work. All public places of socialising such as pubs are in themselves very exhausting. Everything in the chaos is competing for my attention and I find it very hard to deduce what is happening around me, in particular where anybody is in relation to myself. In addition, lip-reading a group of people is very tiring on my eyes. I seem unable to teach myself to hear properly and this causes many problems.

At work and college I have come across many new words which I would like to be able to use. Just from hearing a word spoken in the normal way, I cannot decipher enough of the blurry disorganised sounds to copy them. My spoken vocabulary has always been dependent upon my mother teaching me to pronounce new words and correcting any anomalies in my present vocabulary. She teaches me a new word by breaking it up into its elementary sounds, helps me to pronounce the individual sounds correctly and then assists me in stringing them together to form a word. It can take quite a while for me to master a new word. I am unable to spell the new words from college and work, therefore I cannot even write them down and take them to my mother. I know that other people my age do not have this problem. Is my inability to correctly hear sounds a Dyslexic trait? Can I improve?

Each evening when I return home from work or college it feels as if my brain is going to explode. All day long my brain has been greedily gobbling up and trying to process all the different stimuli. I wish I could switch my brain off and stop it from processing absolutely everything that is around me. It is exhausting, continually processing all the intertwined smells, sounds, tastes, visual things and sensations against my skin. Most of these senses are distorted and give me a misleading impression of 'the world'. At least at home there are not so many stimuli. Consequently my brain has a chance to finish processing all the bombardment from the day. How do other people block out things that are happening around them, in order to concentrate? My father says that everybody must learn to concentrate. The only time I can rest is in bed while I am asleep, this is the only time I escape from the relentless barrage of incoming data from the outside world. The next best place is in the bathroom where nobody disturbs me. Each night I have a bath. This is my time for contemplation of life, the universe and everything. Why do things exist? What is meant by existence? I wish I could understand more about the world.

At work we are being sent on a 'character development' course. It involves camping and orienteering for 4 days in the Lake District. The long coach journey has been extremely exhausting, but before I can go to bed we must erect our tents and each cook ourselves dinner on a portable gas stove. Why does everyone else still have so much energy? Having eaten dinner, I crawl into my sleeping bag and go to sleep. On the first day we are going walking across the hills with the intention of camping out in a cave (without any tents). We will each have to sleep in a large plastic bag! Walking is obviously difficult at the best of times, but trying to carry a big heavy rucksack on my back is a real problem. I need much more control and tension in my muscles to prevent me from falling over. To make matters worse there is a strong wind that is buffeting us and this is making standing upright very hard. We spent all day walking and I was absolutely exhausted by the time we arrived at the cave where we were supposed to camp out over night. My exhaustion had caused me to become very cold and I was in the first stages of hypothermia. As a result, the whole group had to come off the mountain and return to the base camp.

Things did not improve as the week progressed. On the second day we went on another long walk. On the third day we went rafting and 'Canadian' canoeing on a lake. I do not understand. How are the other people coping with the exhaustion and pain? How do they have enough mental stamina to cook themselves food in the evening? Why am I so poor at coping with the pain? By the time the fourth day came I was totally exhausted and in a great deal of pain. Right at the beginning of the day, while 'Gill Walking', I slipped into the river and got very wet! Once we had walked up to the top of the river we then walked to a sheer cliff and abseiled down it. I have absolutely no fear of heights so abseiling down the cliff was easy. I sat on the ground at the bottom of the cliff waiting for the rest of the group to come down the rock face. It was a relief to sit down, as the pain and exhaustion were so overwhelming. I did not realise how low my body temperature was dropping. This is not surprising because even under normal circumstances I have little and sometimes no idea of my body temperature.

A few hours later, when we had arrived back at the campsite, we all went to the local pub. The warmth in the pub overwhelmed me and I collapsed from hypothermia and exhaustion. I have no recall of anything that happened in the next hour, but strangely nobody called a doctor! No one, myself included, can work out why I have become so much more exhausted than everybody else. On my return home, I was sent to see a doctor but he was also unable to explain why a young healthy person should become so exhausted. I wish I could cope with my body as well as everybody else seems to. If only my mind was stronger I could overcome the pain and tiredness like everybody else. (In hindsight, with knowledge of my disability, it is hardly surprising that I became exhausted.)

I am beginning to realise that spending eleven years at school has left me with some unpleasant legacies. Often I feel as if madness is shortly going to consume me. Going mad does not appeal to me, therefore to prevent this, the only logical course of action seems to be to understand myself. I will have to analyse my peculiar reactions to things until I can comprehend what is going on. I know that within my mind there exists an extremely high security prison with many walls and force fields preventing the contents from escaping. The prison exists to safely store all my past negative emotions. At present I am still shovelling ever more things in there and do not know what else to do.

There are other areas of my reactions to things that I believe can be dealt with. For instance, during my secondary school days, if I saw someone I recognised, I always walked off in another direction to avoid trouble. Despite there now being no threat, I have found myself doing the exact same thing at work. Recognising this as a bad behavioural pattern has made me decide to walk past people I know and say 'hello'. This might sound very easy but is in fact very nerve racking and takes a tremendous amount of courage. Another problem is that my self-esteem is virtually non-existent, which results in me behaving in a very quiet and shy manner. If I can eliminate some of the defensive strategies that I have built, I will be in a much better position to appear to behave in a more sociable normal fashion.

A strategy I still need is the one to cope with the illusiveness of time. I have developed a routine which helps give each day and week a structure and meaning relative to time, as follows:-

07:00 Get out of bed	16:00 catch bus home
07:10 Eat breakfast	16:35 Arrive home
07:35 catch bus to work	17:30 Watch television
08:00 Start work	18:00 Eat dinner
12:45 Lunch starts	21:00 Watch daily news on television
13:15 Lunch ends	22:15 Get into bed

I can cope with changes to my schedule but they are resisted because they disorientate me within time. The overall structures in my routines are always complicated. Each type of day has a predefined preferred structure, i.e. college days, workdays, Saturdays, Sundays.

Despite all the enormous difficulties I have experienced throughout this academic year, I achieved merits in all the subjects on the college course. In addition, at work I have managed to successfully complete the first year of my apprenticeship. At last I am beginning to find a way through the Dyslexia and out into the world.

I have never spoken about any of the abuse I received at school until today, since it is obviously my fault for being so slow and stupid. Edna and myself were talking about school and Dyslexia and how many Dyslexic children have a hard time at school, when I happened to very vaguely mention about some of the derision I received. I feel so guilty. Edna has somehow managed to get everything twisted around. For some inexplicable reason she seems to think that it was my abusers that were in the wrong, rather than me. It seems unjust to blame the people who taunted me when it was not their fault. They mocked me because I am such a disastrous excuse for a person. Why does Edna not realise this? Although, it is rather novel that Edna chooses to be on my side! I just hope that when my parents return she does not tell them what I told her, because they do not know what happened at school and if they did they would know it was due to my shortcomings.

I have come to Austria on a holiday with my family. I like Austria, but travelling here was a problem because we flew. After boats, aeroplanes are my worse mode of transport. When in a plane I never know which way is upright. To overcome this I have a drink on the tray in front of me. The top surface of the liquid in the cup will always remain horizontal (because of gravity) and therefore I have a reference and always know which way is upright even when the aeroplane banks round. The other terrible thing about flying is that I get a tremendous pain in my ears during the flight, but especially when taking off and landing.

Now that we have been in Austria several days my ears have recovered from the flight and today I am going on an organised bike ride. I learnt to ride a bike many years ago. The only drawback is that it is painful and of course I topple over if inadequate attention is paid to speed, turning forces and the position of my body relative to gravity.

We have been cycling for a few hours and gently meander our way up the side of a mountain. The group slowly re-congregates at the top of the mountain, while those of us who reached the top first wait for the stragglers. I am going to eat a cheese filled bread roll in order to replace some of my energy. The group leader has a strong accent and is very hard to understand. He is addressing the whole group but I am struggling to decipher any of the words he is saying, so I start sucking a boiled sweet to give me some immediate energy.

We are at last setting off again to descend the mountain. The top of the bike bell has fallen off and is rolling down the road. Stopping, I pick it up and attempt to screw the top back. The group leader stops to see what I am doing but neither of us can replace the bell top. While we are fiddling, everybody else has passed us and after a few minutes we give up and set off again. I need to keep up with the group leader for he is now my only reference and I have no idea of the way back to the hotel from here. We accelerate and continue to accelerate as we descend. I cycle close behind, copying his every move. At last we have started to catch up with some of the people, but they are travelling so much slower than us, that the group leader is still my only feasible reference. Still accelerating we enter a long stretch with a sweeping bend. A sheer cliff reaches up the mountain on the left side of the road and, along the opposite side a stone wall sweeps around the corner, behind which the mountain falls away to the bottom of the valley. Maybe now I can slow down and follow someone else. As I try to apply the brakes the bike just shudders and nothing happens. At this speed and angle of approach to the corner, there is no way I am going to make it round unless I can slow down. Applying the brakes again the bike still shudders and my speed continues to increase. I am heading straight for the stone wall and cannot adjust my course sufficiently to get safely round the corner. Once again I try the brakes. Nothing is happening. The bike shudders as a pedal scores through the ground........too much momentum...elbows on stone wall............

.......falling over wall...........................falling................................

........the world is upside down........falling........falling.................

.............tucking my legs and arms into my body............

...................falling through trees....................

.........................Falling........................

2

....Second year of Electronic Apprenticeship and day release course at college. For most of this academic year I was aged 18....

Yes, I lived! My only injuries were very minor; lacerations to my legs and arms (no permanent scarring), bruises and whiplash. It was only by sheer luck that I was not killed. Apparently around the next corner there was a deep ravine. To have that sort of accident and literally be able to stand up and walk away, must be a chance occurrence. Or is there an entity in the universe, such as a God, who intervened and saved me? Whatever, I have stared death in the face and cheated it. I feel so grateful to be alive that my appetite for suicide has vanished, particularly in the light of my relative success at work and college. Now that I am 18 years old, how can I use my life? I promise myself that I will endeavour not to get into any situation as gruesome as my final years at school. Whatever I am going to do, I refuse to let my past affect my future in a negative way.

It has been brought to my attention that many Dyslexic people may suffer from Scotopic[6] Sensitivity Syndrome, some sort of defect in their vision. The degree of visual defect can be slight or severe and varies from person to person. The standard tests that an Optician performs do not check or pick up these visual-processing distortions. Significant visual distortions will obviously affect reading. This is interesting, because it is claimed that this faulty vision can be corrected by wearing glasses with coloured lenses. Could coloured lenses really make any difference? The concept sounds a bit farfetched. Do I see things differently? If yes, how do other people see? Could faulty vision be the reason why my reading is very poor? I am short-sighted, but glasses correct this. Someone once suggested that the words I see may be processed on the wrong side of my brain, causing them to become unintelligible - does this seem more feasible?

I have been for an assessment for Scotopic Sensitivity Syndrome and it has been confirmed that my vision is indeed very different/defective and that tinted lenses may be helpful. Now I have a chance to try a range of different coloured lenses. Surprisingly, many of the colours actually make aspects of my sight worse. For instance, I see even less on a page of writing or the page appears too bright. It is incredible, this colour is wonderful, everything seems so much clearer and my eyes feel so different; even relaxed? The difference is so marked that this cannot possibly be a placebo effect. A friend had suggested that, if the coloured lenses did indeed improve my vision that I might not like the 'new world', but this is definitely not the case. As a result of this assessment I have been prescribed a pair of glasses with

---

[6] The word Scotopic means; dim light vision when the eyes are dark-adapted, which is considered to be controlled by the rods of the retina. I believe that it is questionable whether the word Scotopic is really the correct word to describe all the different facets of the visual distortions, which come under the general heading of Scotopic Sensitivity Syndrome.

light blue coloured lenses. (I appreciate that from a scientific point of view my interpretation of improvement is not currently measurable and thus the actual physiological/neurological effectiveness of the coloured lenses cannot readily be disproved or for that matter proved!)

For the first time in my life I have experienced a different way of seeing, which has given me a frame of reference to start exploring how other people see. I now realise that what I have been seeing and assumed was clear and not distorted, is by 'normal' standards blurred and distorted. After many long varied discussions with my parents and selected friends, I am slowly beginning to build up a good idea of how 'normal' people see. My conclusions are a revelation to me. 'Normal' people see everything so still and calm, stationary items appear completely still and there are no wild shadows or minute white bits randomly zooming around in a mesmerising chaos. Furthermore, 'normal' people are able to see clearly across a wide scene. Their vision does not start off clear in the very centre of the field of vision and rapidly deteriorate towards the edges. When they look at writing it does not move around and the black lettering is distinctive from the white background.

How do the blue lenses in my glasses help me? In my case they enable me to see a little better but not as well as the average person. It is reported that for some people, the coloured lenses completely cure all visual distortions (I think this relates to people with milder versions of the syndrome). I have noticed the following improvements in my vision:-

* Wider focal vision, there is less discontinuity, often I can see all the letters in a 5 letter word as opposed to two or less. (This narrow focal vision prevents me from seeing and consequentially from visualising whole words, which is why the 'look and say' method was ineffective and why I could not learn to read or spell before I was taught phonetics.)

* Reduced glare and spiky effects from lights or reflected sun. (This effect is like looking through a smeary windscreen, spots of reflected sun on the car in front appear to come out towards me.)

* I can distinguish the 'real' shadows cast across objects.

* Decreased bright shadows around letters and large moving shadows on pages of writing.

* Diminished manic minute white bits. Looking through my eyes is analogous to trying to watch a poorly tuned Television, or looking through a rapidly moving fine mesh that is in front of the eyes.

* Stationary objects appear to move around less.

These improvements have helped me to study for longer periods before becoming fatigued, and to write and copy more accurately. I can now read a book or an article for about 10 to 15 minutes before becoming too tired and losing my concentration. In addition my studying is not so hampered by headaches and aching eyes, because it now takes a little longer for the pain to become overwhelming.

When it is absolutely dark I see a mirage of moving colours in front of my eyes - I have not noticed that this changes while using the coloured lenses. Is this the same effect that astronauts complain of whilst in space? If the absence of gravity upsets their balance systems perhaps this could indicate that my balance system is malfunctioning?

I have attempted to illustrate how I see a page of written text.

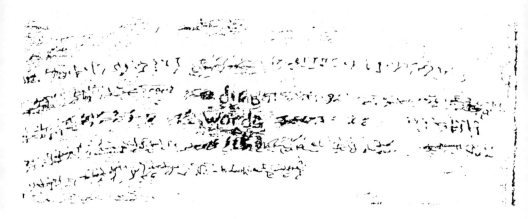

I cannot see the diagram as a whole, but am able to scan my eyes across it to confirm that it is a good representation of my vision. In reality what I see is worse because I see white bits and shadows moving around.

In the context of my work and study my father has been saying for many years that I must learn to concentrate, but as yet I have found no way of keeping my attention on one thing for more than a micro moment. In a noisy and crowded office or classroom the sound and movement around me become intermingled with the task in hand. Even when I am working in a peaceful environment the closest I ever come to concentration is to do my work and at the same time use the rest of my brain to think about other things. In my mind I can alternate very quickly between my work which involves logical thought and the other things which are non-logic based. This gives the false impression of concentration. How do other people concentrate on only one thing at a time? How do other people filter out any external stimuli?

My mother complains that I get stuck in ruts because I tend for weeks on end, to do one type of major activity only. For instance, I study to the exclusion of everything else, or I may build something and will do only that until it is completed. (Whilst writing the main body of this book I did nothing else for six months!) Doing one activity at a time greatly limits the distractions, which means I can better focus my mind on that task. If I attempt to study, design, build, write, all in the same day, for weeks on end I find that all the different things become intertwined and muddled in my mind, until it feels as if it is going to burst.

Noise is one of my worst enemies. It rudely intrudes upon my thought processes. Everywhere there is too much noise. So many machine sounds: cars, aeroplanes, trains, washing machines, fans, etc. My hearing is so acute that even high pitched sound from CRT televisions seems loud. So many people orientated sounds: voices, footsteps, coughing, etc. I cannot escape the sounds, they bombard me all day, everyday. The constant noise drives me crazy and it is frustrating not being able to stop it. Noise can be so mentally painful that sometimes I wish I could go permanently deaf. I long to go somewhere quiet just for a moment, where there is very little or no sound. I just need a rest from noise. But even when it is absolutely quiet I can still hear high pitched buzzing. Why? Is this tinnitus?

Jenny still insists on playing her music while we are both studying and I am unable to persuade her to cut the noise level. My parents and Jenny believe the noise is fairly quiet and that I must tolerate it and learn to concentrate. If Jenny understood the enormous amount of effort I need to put into studying, especially when there is any distraction such as her music, I am sure that she would try to help me, rather than hinder me. I try to give her the benefit of the doubt. Recently, in all situations I have been making a concerted effort to become tolerant of my family and attempt not to become frustrated and irritated when they misunderstand me.

I believe if my parents still misunderstand me, having spent so many years with me, then there is little hope of anyone else comprehending my way of operating. It is acutely painful that those closest to me are unable to understand or accept me for who I am. Their misinterpretation of my intentions must be caused by the inadequate way I express myself.

I have been studying people and their reactions to find out more about the way they behave. The television is a good place to learn about people and how they respond under certain situations. Soap operas are a particularly good place to study emotional responses, because a wide range of different circumstances arises more often than they do in real life. In addition, I have been watching all the interactions of people at work and college. To aid my interaction with 'the world' I am trying to develop a deeper understanding of the English language. To achieve this goal I am asking selected friends and family who are tolerant of my differences, how they would react if I say certain sentences to them. The sentences span a huge range of subject areas.

After many months of asking questions, I am beginning to have a better understanding of the English language and now have more idea of when to use certain words and phrases. However, I have noticed that my selected friends and family are becoming fed up with what they see as a game, consequently my investigations into responses to the English language are once again going to be confined to observation only.

Compared with other people, my understanding seems rather confined to everyday straightforward English. For instance I never appreciate or understand poetic language - it is meaningless. Dad has tried to explain the nuances of language to me but I am unable to grasp what he is trying to tell me. Plus, inaccurate use of language often catches me out. For instance, recently my father came home from work and related a story about the day's events, in which he happened to say,

"... and then Ruth nearly died of laughter....." I was naturally concerned and naively asked,

"What happened, did she need to go to hospital?" This was a bad choice of question. My father was furious. I had apparently ruined the flow of his story and was told that I was more than old enough to know better than to take the English language so literally. I do not understand how to tell the difference between language that tells the truth and the paradox of language that totally misrepresents the facts, but mysteriously implies truth.

This year is just as tough as the first year of my apprenticeship. The older I become the greater my problems seem to be because I am expected to do so much more. As a result my strategies are becoming ever more ingenious and complex. Nobody has ever helped me develop a strategy, they are my own and secret way of dealing with life. I have nearly completed designing a strategy called 'I am not myself'. The successful development of this strategy has been a lifetime's quest. The object of the strategy is to remove my real self from trying to deal with the outside world and to create an artificial personality for myself. This means the real me is separate from what I am doing. The artificial personality is constructed from all the 'best' points I see in other people e.g. consideration, tolerance, approaches for dealing with situations/people, open-mindedness etc. and the moral code of conduct drummed into me as a child and young adult. Using this strategy gives me a frame of reference for communicating with people and enables me to do many things that I would otherwise be unable to cope with, or have the confidence to attempt. The artificial personality is built on a solid foundation of logic, which gives me the ability to behave in a logical way in which there is no room for flaws, such as fear or low self-esteem.

As part of my apprenticeship, every two or three months I have the challenge of changing departments to experience how a different area of the company operates. One problem is that there seems to be a lack of available work for the apprentices. I have an unusual ability for solving practical problems in a lateral manner, which means that I sometimes end up informing fully qualified experienced engineers where they are going wrong! So the fact that there is not much work reduces the possibility of me embarrassing any engineers, which is probably much better for my reputation. A friend has made a very odd suggestion. She says that I should spend the spare time 'learning about people'. I do not really understand what she means. I have never told her that people are unimportant. She also says that I should write a book about my experiences of suffering from Dyslexia, but I am a Dyslexic, I would never write a book! I would be a traitor to my hatred of books. I feel there is something true in what she is saying, but I am not sure what. (For many years her words nagged at me.) However, the lack of work does mean that I sometimes manage to do all my college homework during office hours. This is a huge help. Reducing the amount of time I am working reduces the amount of pain I am in. It is obvious that the location and intensity of pain is a direct result of what a person is doing. I wish I were not so feeble-minded.

Recently I have started playing badminton and am very determined to be a reasonable player. In order to make my body do all of the complex actions related to playing a racket sport, I have designed a new and powerful strategy. This new strategy has been motivated by my inability to learn new skills as quickly as other people. It helps me to learn to control my body and involves using my imagination to conceptualise all the different movements I need and how they should make my muscles feel. So basically I practise my badminton while at home sitting in an armchair! (The strategy soon worked and after about one year of practising I was able to play badminton to a reasonable level, although playing still required an enormous amount of mental effort.)

At college I am making some consistent sense of the symbols used to describe mathematical concepts. One day, most of the people in the class, myself included, were getting in a terrible muddle with some Differential Calculus, partly because we were doing the basic algebra incorrectly. Then the lecturer wrote the most revealing equation on the blackboard; $b + (-c) = b - c$. Now for the first time I understand that it is the figure after the minus sign which is negative. (Up until this point I was unsure whether to subtract b from c or c from b.)

With the help of a friend and the maths lecturer, as the academic year has progressed, I have managed to come to grips with much of the syntax of mathematics. These improvements in my usage of mathematical symbols have been an enormous help to my understanding of many basic aspects of the theories of Electronics. I am still completely unable to do mental arithmetic, despite understanding what must be done, because I invariably forget part of the sum before I can finish it; the numbers get lost, forgotten. It is as if the numbers fall down holes in my mind! When using the calculator I can now anticipate whether the answer to the sum will be large or small. Up until now I have just hoped that my calculations have given me answers of a sensible magnitude. I cannot remember a list of figures over more than a couple of seconds because they get lost in my mind and can never be recalled. This causes particularly irritating problems when looking up a page number in an index. Invariably I need to look up the page number several times because I cannot remember it long enough to find the page! Also when using the calculator I often forget the numbers before I can enter them.

My new found insights into the syntax of mathematics and the secondary effects of the blue lenses (e.g. of reduced tiredness and pain) are having a healthy effect on my college marks. My grades have increased from merits last year, to distinctions this year. At last I have found something that I can excel at. This gives me a sense of purpose. The pain does not seem such a high price to pay when I can actually achieve something worthwhile.

I just wish that I could make equal sense of an analogue clock face and particularly the analogue meters we use at college and work. It is so hard for me to read off a measurement correctly without getting into a muddle. The confusion occurs because I do not have any sense of direction. It is also very hard for me to distinguish between left/right, east/west, up/down, b/d, p/q, clockwise/anticlockwise, past/present/futuristic tenses (hence the style in which this book is written!) and anything else which is symmetrical. To help overcome this I use mnemonics and recognise the minor scars on my hands that enable me to differentiate between them. (My watch is always worn on my left wrist). I guess this confusion is somehow caused by Dyslexia. Why am I Dyslexic? Why me?

Jenny knows many people and has many friends. I know relatively few people and equally have comparably few friends. This does not really bother me since nobody understands me. If the truth were known the best friend I have ever had is my computer. Unlike humans, my computer acts in a logical and consistent fashion.

My parents seem to notice my lack of social activity and find it a bit odd. Often they pass comments such as; why do you not go out more? Or why do you not join in with any of the social activities at work, college etc.? (Unbeknown to me, my mother was becoming quite worried about my lack of social interaction.) I have worked out the best compromise possible within my energy limitations. One evening of the week is spent at college and another playing badminton. At the weekend, one night is spent at a local pub with one or two friends and the other night is spent with a small Youth Group. Each night I must be in bed by 22.15 and get up in the morning no earlier than 07.00. This way I have just enough energy without becoming completely exhausted. If one night I go to bed a quarter or half an hour later than usual, I unfortunately, always seem to suffer for it the next day. Why do I become so much more tired than other people? There is no apparent medical reason. It is not that I would not like more friends but rather that people drain my valuable energy resources. They want to talk and/or go out and all these things I enjoy, but the cost on my energy levels is very high, too high.

3

....Third, and final year of Electronic Apprenticeship. First year of HNC day release course at college. For most of this academic year I was aged 19....

Success...Success. It's marvellous, I have found something that I am very good at. I achieved straight distinctions in my final and second year of the BTEC National Certificate in Electronic Engineering, with an average mark of 91%. The college have just awarded me the 'Best Student of Engineering in 1987-1988'. My perseverance has paid off. It seems like a fairy-tale, after all this time I have truly made it to the top in something. Just over two years ago, when my secondary school days had finished, many with whom I came into contact, considered me to be very unintelligent, but now nobody treats me as if I am a dimwit.

Two years ago, when I reluctantly started the BTEC National Certificate course at college, I had intended it to be the final academic course I ever took. However, in the light of my recent academic success I have decided to carry on and obtain a BTEC Higher National Certificate (HNC) in electronic engineering. If I maintain high marks through the HNC course, maybe I could go to University and do an Honours Degree. I subtly suggested this to my mother to test her opinion of my intellectual ability, but discovered that she felt that I was definitely not clever enough to go to University. Is she right? To do the HNC I have to change to a College of Higher Education.

At this college of Higher Education the lecturers cover the subject matter even faster than at the previous college. This is no longer a problem because I now have a deep enough understanding of Electronics and Mathematics to somehow instinctively know what most of the next stages are. Sometimes my insight surprises the lecturers and also my colleagues at work. Therefore, the lectures very often simply confirm and refine my hypotheses, which makes doing this course much easier. In all aspects of life I try to anticipate a range of possibilities of what is about to happen next. This enables me to keep up with people rather than being the usual one step behind. For example, if I know what someone is likely to say next, I do not need to worry about trying to hear or lip-read every word. The newly adapted anticipation strategy is becoming very powerful, so much so that I am often several steps ahead of the people around me. I wonder if other people use this strategy?

Unfortunately, even now, my Dyslexia makes it extremely difficult for me to effectively do any filing, form filling or any paper work. But more frustratingly my Dyslexia still impedes my usage of the English language, I have not yet found a way to express most of my thoughts. For the most part I seem unable to penetrate 'the world' of language and expression. Despite desperately wanting to express myself, words completely elude me. Occasionally, some of my less advanced thoughts find their way through the barrier and out into 'the world' of language.

It is as hard for me to communicate with 'the world' as it is correctly to interpret. One thing, which is very unnerving, is when I am in a room at home and I see a person standing or walking, when there is no actual person there. I do not know what causes these optical illusions at the peripheries of my vision, but they are enough to drive a person insane. These optical illusions often happen, but it is only when I know there is nobody around that they are disconcerting. Sometimes when I am at home on my own, suddenly out of the corner of my eye, I see someone walking past the door of the room that I am in. When this happens my blood runs cold and I always need to walk out of the room and convince myself that there is nobody there. In a crowded area there is so much chaos that it would be virtually impossible to distinguish the illusions from reality. How do other people cope with these mirages? Or is this some sort of schizophrenic problem? Am I seeing real ghosts? Am I going insane?

My inability to behave in a 'normal' fashion is frustrating. I cannot exactly put my finger on what is wrong, but something is definitely not right. My interpretation of life has always been so different from that of the people around me. There could be two possible reasons for this, either I am different from everybody else or I am completely hopeless at coping. Since I have no evidence to suggest that there is anything wrong with me other than Dyslexia, I must assume that I am just hopeless at coping. For example, I find stepping onto an escalator or walking down a very noisy road difficult and sometimes frightening. Either other people do not have these fears, or I am much worse at suppressing them. Whichever is true, I must be psychologically infirm, therefore must do my best to cover up my psychological inadequacies.

I have written a short report to help people understand the way I see. So far it has helped my parents, my friends, colleagues at work and a college lecturer understand me a little better. I feel that the more people I can educate about Dyslexia and the associated problems of defective vision, the greater chance there is that people suffering from Dyslexia will understand more about themselves and will be better understood by those around them. I realise that educating the small number of people I come into contact with, is infinitesimal compared with all the people in the world, but it is a start.

Understanding the syntax of the mathematical symbols has opened up a whole new world to me. For the first time I am now able to express some of my mathematical thoughts and have been communicating at a closer level to my thought processes. This is an absolutely wonderful breakthrough. I have also discovered that if text is on dull coloured paper it further improves my vision, the writing appears clearer. There is a particular brand of blue coloured A4 writing paper that I now use at college, as this increases my chances of seeing what I am doing. I just wish I could see the whole of an equation simultaneously.

Am I clever enough to attend university to do an Honours Degree in engineering? This question has been going through my mind for weeks and weeks, but I do not have the courage to ask the lecturer at college in case the answer is 'no'. One day the lecturer completely unexpectedly said,

"Have you ever considered the possibility of going to university?" I cannot believe my luck because this saves me from broaching the subject! To even bother to ask the question the lecturer must believe that it is a feasible possibility. This is wonderful. If it was possible for me to study at university I could concentrate on my studies rather than try to juggle college and work. After a short discussion I decided that this was definitely what I wanted to do. (At this point in time I was simply perceived as intelligent, severely dyslexic, suffering from some eyesight problems and having overcome the difficulties!)

There is something that still eludes me. It all started the other day at college. The whole class was doing a mathematical example on 'Hysteresis Loops' in which we needed to convert cubic centimetres into cubic metres. This seemed to be an easy task, since 50cm equals 0.5m it follows that 50cm3 must equal 0.5m3! I seem unable to obtain the correct answer and the lecturer has told me to think about the method that I have used to convert from centimetres to metres. But surely 50cm3 must equal 0.5m3. Perplexed I asked,

"How else would anyone convert centimetres to metres?". Fortunately the lecturer was patient and he wrote on my paper: 1 000 000cm3 = 1m3.

"I do not understand how that can possibly be correct", I replied. After some further discussion the lecturer went to his office and returned with some 'dice' to demonstrate the principal that a cubic unit (e.g. m3) takes up three-dimensional space. Equally, it emerged that a square unit (e.g. m2) takes up two-dimensional space. This is a revelation to me but I find this impossible to visualise and can only imagine it on an abstract level. I view and imagine the world as a set of edges or lines. Let me briefly explain; to comprehend a square I would think of four straight lines forming a closed loop and with each line joined to the next with an internal angle of 90o. This same principle extends for comprehending three-dimensional space. All this raises some interesting questions; 'Do I see in three dimensions?', 'Do I perceive in my mind's eye in three dimensions?', 'Does my brain merge the images from my eyes in the correct way?'. I strongly suspect the answer to these questions is 'no', but I have no solid frame of reference on which to confirm my hypothesis.

I am very ashamed of my Dyslexia and never wish to draw any attention to it.

"Alison, it is not your fault that you are Dyslexic", commented the lecturer. That comment has taken me by surprise. Almost without realising it I have always blamed myself for being Dyslexic. Yes, I see it now, it cannot possibly be my fault. I never did anything to deserve to be Dyslexic. Dyslexia is just one of those things which some people are unfortunately afflicted with, without it being anybody's fault. It is simply one of the potential hazards of owning a human body. It is like a great weight has been lifted off my shoulders. The shame and guilt have gone.

The lecturer took me by surprise again by saying that my experiences at school could have so easily caused me to become bitter and twisted. My logic replied,

"There is no point in being bitter and twisted." Hang on a minute, if it is not my fault that I am Dyslexic then why has everybody treated me so badly? For the first time I am beginning to feel an uncontrollable anger towards those people who have hurt me. What were they thinking about? Why did my parents and teachers treat me as if I was brainless? I must try and quash this anger before I really do start to become bitter.

At work, my apprenticeship has nearly finished. The anxiety of whether any department in the company would offer me a job has now vanished. I have passed a job interview to enter one of the departments. It is the department that I most enjoyed being in while I was doing my apprenticeship. I am now a trainee Repair, Test & Calibration Engineer. On the face of it, everything seems to be going so well for me. Again this year, like last, I have achieved Distinctions in all the subjects at college, which is fabulous and to the best of my knowledge I have again achieved the highest average mark on the course. My average mark this year is 93%. It feels very strange and somehow wrong being at the top after lying at the bottom for the whole of my school life. Now that my parents have accepted that I am fairly bright we are looking into the possibility of me going to university.

I am paying the penalty for my lifestyle. My social life is much the same as it has been for a long while. Why do I get so weary? Why is it, the more I do the worse the pain becomes. The pain is now even worse than it was while I was at school because I now have to work for much longer hours. This lifestyle is draining me, wearing me out. I need a long rest, my brain is going to burst, and I am so very tired. What is the point of me using up all my energy at work and then having virtually none left for any social activities? It is so frustrating having such limited energy. What sort of life am I living?

SIX

Confrontation

1

....*September 1989. Fourth and final year of day release course at college. I start my first job having completed the apprenticeship in Electronic Engineering. For most of this academic year I was aged 20....*

For many years, I have believed that the neurological make up of the brain of a Dyslexic person is somehow different, but exactly what causes these differences has never been clear to me. It is very often considered that the problem is initially caused by a 'faulty' part in a gene or is a genetic tendency. So it has come as rather a surprise to learn that there may be a possible explanation and even cure which could correct the neurological behaviour of the brain! If I can be cured it would be miraculous. My parents have always told me that I must overcome my problems and live in the 'real' world. How can the neurological pathways around the brain be changed? This all seems a bit far-fetched. However, I am intrigued and wish to find out more.

My search for a true understanding of Dyslexia has begun in earnest. Little did I know at this time, but my search was to bring me to an understanding of many things far beyond the realms of 'just simple' Dyslexia. The particular theory, which I am presently investigating, suggests to me that there are developmental reflexes that should develop in the central nervous system before birth and in the first one to two years of life. As far as I understand, a lack of development in the reflexes can cause mild to severe problems, depending upon where and how many of these reflexes are defective. It has been intimated that this could be the cause of some of my problems and that following a specially designed exercise programme could help my reflex problems, which in turn would improve my co-ordination and balance. There were some inescapable facts that came to light:-

My balance is very poor, as are all aspects of my coordination and fine muscle control. My fine eye muscle control is not functioning properly and it appears that I have some sort of visual perceptual problems. My hearing is affected because my brain seems unable to sort out all the sounds. On top of all this, my body is muscularly tense because I need to physically hold it together. Most importantly there does not seem to be any defect in my psychology, which could have distorted the above findings, thus my inability to do many things is purely a physical problem.

My open-minded local GP (doctor) suggested that provided the treatment did not make me any worse and did not have debilitating side effects, there was no real harm in trying the exercises which are purported to correct/improve the central nervous system's operation. My attitude towards this very unusual form of treatment is; if it works that is brilliant, if it partly works that is good, if it makes no difference I have not lost anything by trying. Is there a definite connection between underdeveloped reflexes and Dyslexia?

Before my parents and I investigated the possibility of my reflexes being underdeveloped, my parents had no idea of the extent of my physical difficulties. The possibility of my reflexes being different has prompted us to discuss how we do and see various things. My parents began to realise that their world was quite different to mine (with respect to physical movements and sight and hearing). Equally, I was surprised to learn how much physically harder many things were for me. We have come to the conclusion that my problems are fairly extensive. It has also emerged that my father has to a lesser degree, some of the problems that I have. For the first time in his life and much to his relief, he now realises that his lack of coordination, concentration and fine muscle control, together with his inability to quickly determine left from right and to read quickly, is not an intellectual inadequacy, but a real physical fault in his neurological make-up. In addition, all the frustration he felt as a child, bad at sports and slow at learning to read, was exactly the same as other people with similar problems. Even as an adult the frustrations continued. He wondered why he could not read as fast as his colleagues at work and why he could not learn to concentrate as well as other people.

Knowledge can be a dangerous thing. I now believe that there are very good neurological reasons for my failing to be 'normal'. I feel a tremendous anger and bitterness towards the people who have unjustly hurt me: family, friends, teachers, classmates, etc. My new found awareness of my situation makes me wonder why I suffer, when all the people I know live comparatively easy lives? Why everybody treated me so badly when it was not my fault? Why nobody realised that my problems were caused by neurological differences rather than psychological inadequacies? I feel completely alone. I do not know anybody else like me. What is the point of living a life, which will be fraught with difficulties, just because my central nervous system operates differently? Why me? Could I complete a university degree despite my difficulties?

My heart is set on attending university and completing an Honours Degree course in Electronic Engineering. Once and for all, I need to establish for myself whether I am clever or not. If I could go to university I would be able to escape the turmoil and stresses of living in the parental home. I would be free. My life would be much easier without my family hassling me.

The universities require that HNC students like myself should achieve straight distinctions. At present I am in my second and final year of my HNC so if I am to have any chance of going to university I must obviously continue achieving distinctions. Having chosen the universities I would like to attend, my mother on my behalf filled in the mountains of associated paperwork. In due time the universities responded and I went for the interviews. To my great surprise, the first university I visited straight away offered me an unconditional place on their course, despite the fact that I had not finished my HNC and therefore did not yet have the usual required entry qualifications. As time progressed, of the universities I applied to, all except one offered me unconditional entry onto their respective courses. As far as I could ascertain the interviewer at the university that did not offer me an unconditional place, seemed strangely worried that all females were liable to develop a phobia about electricity and consequently be unable to complete the course!

While my quest for a place at a university is going extremely well, the rest of my life is falling to pieces. For over six years I have been working to my absolute limits, perhaps even beyond my capacity, under very difficult circumstances in which nobody understands me. Physical and emotional exhaustion is building up and overcoming me. In many areas of my life, on the surface things are much better, my parents attitude towards me is much improved. I am doing fine at work, well at college and have potential university places waiting for me. All these things give me great pleasure and a sense of self-worth. So why do I feel so worn out?

At present I am still spending one day (9am - 8:30pm) a week at college and the four remaining days at work. I am desperately trying to juggle my college work and new job, and no longer have the opportunity to do any college work during office hours. As a result my college work has fallen behind. When I return home from work my energy level is extremely low, so much so that my college work takes me considerably longer than usual. At the weekends I try to recuperate but 2 days is not enough. The demands and expectations of having a job are far greater than they were when I was a mere apprentice. Under this light, university is an attractive option because it would be easier to achieve a degree on a full-time basis rather than the present part-time basis.

The older I become the more things I am expected to be able to do. This is a problem, because pain and tiredness, which are a result of what I am doing, make appearing reasonably normal, difficult. As the years progress being acceptably normal is like an unattainable goal which keeps moving further away and although I make progress I seem unable to reach it. How do other people manage to keep up with the demands of everyday living? At the end of each day my mind is a swirling muddle as I try to process all that has happened and is happening around me.

My appetite to be normal is fast disappearing. For some years now I have been using a strategy which I created called 'I am not myself' which uses a superficial, artificial personality and shields the real me from 'the world'. After relying on the strategy for so many days, weeks and years, I have completely forgotten who I really am. I need to re-discover the real me and am therefore dismantling the strategy. This is my own personal struggle, nobody in the whole world knows about my artificial personality. Dismantling it could be dangerous because I will have to cope with all my real emotions and feelings, but hopefully now that I am older this will be easier. I must rely on my logic and memory of past experience to decide how to react at each moment in time.

During the college year I fell very behind with my college work. The exercise programme, which was supposed to be helping my co-ordination and balance, had added to my tiredness and I was able to hide behind it and blame it for all my overall tiredness. This meant that in the short term there was an obvious reason for my tiredness, which anyone could understand. In order to catch up, so that I could safely go to university without being behind, I resigned from my job. The company refused my resignation and put me on unpaid leave but still generously offered to sponsor me if I went to university.

My endeavours to catch up were based on my ability to understand and remember most things, after reading them only once. For me there is a very fine line between doing very well and failing. Either I have or have not read the material. In addition, because of my problems with reading, I only ever read a very limited amount. I would never contemplate reading a whole chapter of a textbook, let alone the whole book. Ideally I need to acquire written information by being read to, either by a person, audio cassettes or a computer. Unfortunately none of these ways are currently available to me. Thankfully I did catch up with all the exams and assignments before the end of the academic year and my end of year marks still averaged 91% and therefore I have obtained distinctions in all my subjects and for this achievement the college gave me an award.

During this summer I would like to have a complete rest to recuperate, to put me in a good and fresh frame of mind, ready for the start of my university life. Unfortunately I seem unable to convey this to my parents and they have very different ideas. My mother has arranged for me to do some voluntary work at a local home for people with severe learning difficulties. I am to work in conjunction with the maintenance team doing practical jobs around the site. The work and people are fine; the only problem is that my opportunity for a really good rest has completely vanished. The only favourable aspect is that I only work mornings, which has been made possible by me claiming that I need to study some more mathematics before going to university. It is true that studying mathematics in further depth would be beneficial, but after working all morning my energy level is too low to concentrate. How will I ever survive the university course if I am so tired at the start of the term?

2

....The first year at university studying for an honours degree in Electronic Engineering. For most of this academic year I was aged 21. By this time I had completely eradicated the strategy 'I am not myself' and no longer used any form of artificial personality. The following pages are constructed using mostly material which I wrote at the time....

My parents have unpacked all my things and left me alone in this small long narrow room, in the middle of a massive block of student accommodation on the mind-boggling university campus. I am now truly alone. There are rooms above, below, to the left, and to the right of me. I am surrounded. There is so much unfamiliar confusion in all the different noises that penetrate the walls of this room. The only way out of this room to the outside world is via a narrow corridor. I find it difficult to walk along the corridor without banging into one wall and then the other. It is as if the corridor shrinks and moves as I walk along it. If anyone sees me they will probably think I am drunk! The campus is a huge maze with many intertwined paths and corridors. Will I ever find the hidden consistency in this labyrinth?

Whilst addressing the whole assembly of first year students, one of the university staff told us that we are not alone and that any problems we may have will not be unique. Also we were told that the university had a great many students pass through it over the years and staff are accustomed to all the problems which could arise. I wish this could be true for me. This statement has made me realise my isolation, nobody here will have come across someone like me. I feel the paradox of being alone in a crowd. I understand that people with reflex problems rarely manage to achieve the required qualifications for entry into university, let alone attempt an honours degree. In fact I can find no past case histories of anyone like myself going to university and completing the course. At least if nothing else the university will realise the difficulties caused by severe dyslexia. But I suppose there is really very little practical help they can offer me on that front.

There is a sense in which I feel my presence here is somehow wrong. I am supposed to be unintelligent, yet I am at one of the top universities in the country. The people who are here with me are equivalent to those who mocked me at school. Students and lecturers alike use such advanced English, that often I have very little idea of what they are talking about. Even now I have difficulty with words such as to/from, back/front, in/out, on/off. For instance, I am still perplexed by phrases such as 'a wind is named from the direction from which it comes'. My comprehension and vocabulary are far too limited and my general knowledge is comparatively poor.

After only a few weeks of university life I am coming up against severe problems. The course is so tiring. There is so much writing and reading to be done. The majority of the reading I need to do is from the blackboards, and OHPs[7] and work sheets, but it is difficult to copy writing or diagrams from either an OHP projection or a blackboard. Fortunately I never have to read more than a few paragraphs out of any textbook.

One of my worst problems is there are so many things to remember to do and get done within a specific time frame. Forward planning which involves time is extremely difficult since I have no sense or 'feeling' of my place in time or for the passing of time in terms of seconds, minutes or hours. On an intellectual level I

---

[7] Over Head Projector (OHP)

understand the passing of time, as a measure of change! The earth rotates once per day and around the sun once every (approx.) 365.25 days, thus the earth changes position relative to the sun. For instance, if I know that I must go to a lecture in one hour's time, I have no idea how soon the hour will be up and no notion of what I can get done in an hour. This means that I am expending much mental effort just keeping track of time so that I arrive everywhere punctually.

Yet another big problem is the noise in the accommodation block where I am living. It is distracting me so badly, that all tasks are taking many times longer to complete. Everything mingles together in my mind: sounds, smells, sights, my work, etc. How can anyone concentrate in this chaos? How is it possible? Perhaps my brain lacks a chemical? Perhaps in 'normal' people, when concentrating, they have a chemical released in the brain, controlled in some way by the sub-conscious, which dulls the senses which are unrelated to the task (e.g. the person's hearing is suppressed when a person is reading, thus irrelevant sound does not disturb them.) If only I could cut out all the external distractions and do my work.

To add to my problems, the sun comes streaming through the window, the brightness is blinding and very long spikes of sunlight come out towards me from places where the sun hits shiny surfaces. Everywhere I go there is the dreaded fluorescent tube lighting. Both sunlight and fluorescent tube lighting increase the rate at which my eyes become tired and augment all my visual distortions (e.g. there are many more little white bits flying around). Spending more than about half an hour under fluorescent lighting gives me a headache and eye ache. My ideal after dark lighting is from 'Daylight'[8] bulbs and during the daylight hours I like natural light which comes through a north-facing window. The carpet and duvet cover in my study room is highly patterned. This causes me to see a whirling mesmerizing mess, which hurts my eyes. The patterns are hard to escape in this small room. Any highly contrasting pattern is a problem. For instance, trying to have a conversation with someone who is wearing a black and white striped shirt is almost impossible. The pattern appears to be jumping around in a mesmerizing fashion and can cause my vision to go fuzzy and remain fuzzy long after the pattern is out of sight.

Knowing my senses transmit unreliable information about my environment makes it easier for me to compensate. I find it requires a great deal of self discipline to be neat and tidy when my perceptions of 'the world' are chaotic and disorganised, paradoxically it is essential to be organised if I am ever to cope with life. I unravel the chaotic information from my senses and brain, using a subtle combination of logic and probability. There are numerous examples, such as; if I recognise someone, I need to decide whether it is likely that the person in question could be in a given place. So if I think I see a friend who works and lives in my home village, when I am 200 hundred miles away at university, I would deduce that it is improbable that the person is on the university campus. I use these same principles

---

[8] Daylight bulbs emit light, which has a similar spectral pattern to that of natural daylight, and are often used by people wishing to do interior photography (e.g. portraits) or needlework after dark.

across all that I see, hear and sense, to enable me to discover the truth about 'the world'.

I can compensate against all the disturbances caused by my faulty neurological make-up and adjust my life around the tiredness. These things I can just about cope with. But the one thing I cannot control or escape from is the pain, which is pushing me over the edge. Everything I do results in pain. This happens because the pain is caused by muscle tension and my compensating for my poorly working central nervous system causes the muscle tension. For instance, if I wish to write down something legible on a piece of paper, I must brace my whole body and eyes and force my arm and hand to make the pen write the letters. If my writing is unreadable, it tends to defeat the object of writing! The longer I hold my body and arm under control, the greater the pain becomes. The principle of pain verses activity applies across all aspects of my daily living. Some instances of this are: eating makes my arms hurt (e.g. cutting up food), sitting in a chair makes my legs and back ache, standing still makes my legs stiff and painful, hanging out washing makes my neck and eyes very painful,..., the list is endless!

Somehow I can not really imagine what it would be like to be able to see, read, write, walk, sit etc. without any pain. Every time I do anything I need to inflict pain upon myself. If humans did not suffer pain they would not have a warning that something was wrong, so I suppose that pain needs to exist. So what is wrong with pain? Basically it prevents me from concentrating and doing things. A friend once said 'mental/emotional pain is worse than physical pain'. I would dispute that. In my experience, extreme pain of either sort is equally torturous and incapacitating, but both sorts of pain simultaneously are mind-blowing. Am I damaging my body by putting it under such extreme tension?

The overall exhaustion means that because I need so much rest, I can only do academic work. The undesirable result is that my social life is non-existent. I vaguely know some of the people in my corridor and know one or two people on my course, but nobody else. What is life all about? Am I living or just existing? How should I cope when my world is so different that nobody ever has much chance of understanding it? How should I cope when 'my world' is not compatible with 'the world'? It is agony having nobody to talk with or bounce ideas off. The vast majority of my thoughts and ideas are, and have always, been locked up in my wordless world in which there is an infinite void between my thoughts and 'the world' of language?

The only way I can deal with this torture is to build a wall of logic, build a mental strategy for coping with 'the world', ensuring that all the frustration and hurt are locked away where they, I hope, will never escape. After many years of this, what will it do to me? The only way to continue seems to be to build ever-stronger strategies and a firmer conviction to logic and also to build sturdier, bigger walls to house all the years of pent-up frustration, emotion, fear and pain. I hope that the strategies never fail and the walls in the mind do not burst. Beyond the wall of logic and strategies is a person bursting to get out, squashed by strategies and folded by logic.

I hope that tomorrow will be no worse than today and since tomorrow is as yet unspoilt, maybe finally my life will be easier. However, there is no logical reason why my life should be suddenly better tomorrow. If my hope runs out it will be a silent goodbye. My quality of life seems to be very poor. I have severe doubts about the wisdom of continuing on here at university.

> What is the point?
> What am I trying to prove?
> How much longer can I keep fighting?
> Tired of fighting?
> Am I starting to lose the fight?
> Have I attempted too much?
> But what would I do with my life if I do not complete the course?
> Can I go somewhere quiet, where there is nobody?
> Is my thirst for knowledge too great to leave university?
> I am losing the power to stay awake?
> Is there a reason to live?

After struggling on for one and a half terms, my mother and Edna came to visit me. They saw that there was no way that I would be able to carry on, because I was so desperately tired and as a result was falling behind with my work. Thankfully I managed to arrange with the university that I should go home and recuperate, while they kept open my place on the course. I spent the rest of the academic year recuperating at home.

I am lost within my frustration of failure to cope with university life. I thought if I escaped to university, life would be much better, away from the hassles of home, but I have discovered that I cannot escape from myself. Time to reflect. Why me? What did I ever do to deserve this affliction? Will I ever find a niche in life? Will I ever be able to effectively communicate in words? I wish that I could communicate. I wish someone could understand me. What can I do to become a 'real' person who is able to interact and join in life's rich tapestry of activities?

SEVEN

Building Bridges

1

...September 1991. Year away from university spent at home resting. For most of this academic year I was aged 22....

For the last two years I have been undertaking an exercise programme which aims to improve the way my central nervous system operates. During this period I have experienced very slight improvements in aspects of my hearing, sight and fine muscle control. However, all these improvements seem to be very unstable. My handwriting speed has increased. My hearing is sometimes a little clearer and the sounds reach my brain in less of a muddle, so are easier to decipher. My vision occasionally becomes marginally clearer, when this happens I can see more of a person's face and birds opening their wings as they flutter from branch to branch. Without the clearer vision it looks as if the birds literally spring from branch to branch!

Once in a while I have the sense of seeing in three dimensions as opposed to my normal two-dimensional vision. When I am seeing in two dimensions everything seems flat and equidistant and there is no natural way of determining where any object is in relation to another object, or myself. Ironically, when I see in three dimensions, I am completely unable to judge distances, but why? 'Normal' people seem to manage. Some things look as if they are bursting forth into my face and other things seem to be receding and falling away from my feet. This is petrifying. The experience of three-dimensional vision has enabled me, for the first time in my life, to visualise three-dimensional space in my mind. I can spin and manipulate images within my imagination in any way that pleases me. Previously and unbeknown to me, before seeing in three dimensions, I only ever imagined things in two dimensions (i.e. flat).

Suddenly perceiving sights and sounds differently is exciting but also extremely frightening. It is like being instantaneously thrust, without any warning, into life on an another planet. As I was unaware that these enhancements were a possible outcome of the exercise programme, the argument that they were purely a placebo is invalid. There are questions that still remain unanswered in my mind, such as; could these improvements have happened anyway as part of some latent development? Why are the improvements so unstable? Within several weeks of returning to university all the improvements vanished! In order to try and attain permanent improvements, I have decided to take a whole year out of university and to purely concentrate on discovering whether it is possible to make my central nervous system work better. Although I believe this is the most sensible way forward it feels as if life is passing me by. I am 22 and have not yet completed one whole year of the degree course, let alone finished it. It seems unfair that my friends and acquaintances have all completed their degree courses, whereas I have barely started.

My rare experience of variations in the operation of my central nervous system, caused by the exercise programme, gives me a frame of reference on which to start an in depth study of how 'normal' people perceive and operate. Hopefully this will enable me to comprehend myself and deduce where I am in relation to 'normal' people. I need to answer the questions; 'Exactly what are my problems?' and 'How can I overcome them more effectively?' The answers to such questions will be particularly useful if it turns out to be impossible for my central nervous system to work properly. The answers should enable me to develop more efficient strategies and compensations.

While I am not working or studying I obviously have many hours of spare time. This has given me the chance to start playing the flute again, although it is taking me longer than I expected to rediscover a good technique for creating a reasonable sound. There is a very small group of musicians at a local church who have invited me to play with them. Since I have nothing better to do this seems like a good opportunity, providing they do not try and brainwash me with religion! Playing on my own at home is easy, but playing with a group is creating problems. It is difficult for me to read the notes from the music, let alone read the timing. To make matters even worse, it is very hard for me to pick out the rhythm. Even a mechanical clock does not seem to tick with constant speed or volume. Once I have picked out the beat it is extremely difficult to judge when to come in. I always come in a fraction of a beat too late. Is there a delay in sound reaching my mind and therefore am I hearing everything later than everybody else? Or does it take me a relatively long time to send the correct messages to my body, so much so that I can never come in at the right moment?

Similarly, in group discussions or during telephone conversations it is hard for me to engage in conversation because I cannot judge when to speak, I am somehow unable to speak at the right time, which results in me butting in or talking at the same time as someone else. This can be compounded by the fact that I find it very hard to hold thoughts in my mind while interpreting what someone else is saying or doing. Sometimes I have to speak my thoughts before I forget them. Language can be so slow and arduous that I find myself answering questions before the person has finished asking the question.

I have always fancied doing some watercolour paintings and now that I have the time, my parents have kindly given me the appropriate paints and paper as a Christmas present. All I have to decide now is what to paint! Up until today I have felt completely uninspired. Today I am in the depths of depression because I am bored and frustrated with living at home. It feels as if there is no point in carrying on. My life seems to lack direction and quality. If my central nervous system cannot be made to work in a more 'normal' fashion how can I realistically return to university? Worse still, nobody understands me. At best I am perceived as 'a bit different'. I find it most disheartening that most people I know, at sometime or another have called me a 'freak' and then said 'you know I did not really mean it in a nasty way'! Being called a freak makes me feel even more isolated and after all it is true that nobody I know has ever come across anybody else like myself. I feel completely alone in the world. What is the point of carrying on?

To try and take my mind off my solitude, I have decided to paint a sunset, using some of my photographs as references. On rare occasions I do pencil sketches, but this also takes a great deal of effort to make the pencil do exactly what I want. I will guess how to mix the paints and apply them to the paper. I would never do anything rash, like read a book on the subject! In order to control my paintbrush I need to brace my whole body. Painting seems to be even harder on my body than drawing. After spending the whole day painting, my body feels like it has been run over by a 'double-decker' bus!

When my parents returned home from work they were amazed at the quality of my painting, especially as I had never been taught or even shown. This has again given me a glimmer of self-worth. Being at home all day does not do much for my already very low self-esteem. Perhaps I am not completely useless after all. (Up until the time of writing this book, I have only painted 3 more pictures, because of the extraordinarily high cost in pain and tiredness.)

By observation and asking people careful questions, I have discovered that people who see in three dimensions can automatically judge distance, they can just see where things are in relation to each other and themselves, and therefore they have 'spacial awareness'. In my two dimensional world, judging distance is achieved by using parallax[9] effects and objects of known sizes (e.g. a door) a technique I developed at Secondary School. For instance, on going for the first time into an ordinary room in an average house, I can obtain a rough idea of space and distance by using objects such as doors, as a reference of size. I can also see how objects apparently move in relation to each other as I walk around the room (i.e. utilise parallax effects). However, if I walk into a garden which I have never visited before, where there would normally be no objects of a known size, it is that much more difficult to judge distance. There is no way of accurately anticipating how large a plant or a tree might be. It is like asking the rhetorical question 'how long is a piece of string?'!

My lack of spacial awareness causes many problems on both the small and large scale. On a small scale it causes difficulties such as judging the edge of a piece of paper. Often I may reach the very edge of the paper whilst half way through a

---

[9] Parallax, is the apparent difference in position or direction of an object as the observer moves. For instance, if you are travelling along in a car and you look out of a side window at two trees, one in the distance and one close to the road, the two trees will appear to move in relation to each other.

word. In addition, I find it extremely hard to draw a picture or diagram to a reasonable size and position on a page. On the large scale it causes difficulties such as; judging speed of traffic (all young children are unable to do this), knowing where the edge of the pavement is, judging where a person is if they are walking alongside me (I persistently walk into the person or across their path), judging when to walk on and off an escalator. In my case, my lack of spacial awareness means that I have no fear of heights. How can I be scared when I have no natural way of telling how far away the ground is?!

I find it completely impossible to focus on a narrow edge, for example a piece of paper or blinds (vertical or venetian). I wish my parents did not have such blinds across our windows at home. If I view any narrow edge such as those mentioned, I have no way of determining it's distance and it feels as if the narrow edge is cutting into my eyes. The excruciating pain makes me instinctively look away. A researcher once suggested that perhaps narrow edges cause an overload somewhere in the visual processing parts of my brain. For me, looking at a narrow edge is like a normal person trying to keep their eyes open if something is moving very fast straight towards them. The instinctive defence is to shut one's eyes. Likewise, when I see a narrow edge, my instinctive reaction is to shut my eyes or look away. I have found it very hard to communicate this problem to my parents, they think I am just being awkward.

It has taken me years to find the words and a frame of reference on which to describe how dreadful shopping is for me. Many ordinary people find shopping tiring but for me it is exhausting and a great strain. Just getting to a shop is bad enough. Travelling in the car, trying to compensate for the disorientating motion, all the trees and lamp posts rushing towards me, the smell of traffic fumes, the overwhelming smell of my mother's perfume, sound of engines whining, is exhausting. Walking along a pavement trying to avoid moving obstacles such as people, trying to keep concentrating on what I am doing so that I do not walk off the pavement or into any other stationary obstacles. All the sounds, smells and sights are all trying to get my attention, causing a confusing blurry mess. Crossing the road is difficult, trying to accurately judge the speed and distance of the traffic, using both my eyes and ears. I have no real sense of which way is upright, so it is important to keep a good vertical reference in sight so that I do not fall over. If loud vehicles come along the road, the level of the sound overloads my brain, causing further deterioration in my sight. If there is a very loud noise my sight may disappear for a moment.

In a shop there are so many sounds, smells and sights all competing for my attention. There may be highly patterned carpets, stripes from vertical blinds, clothes and packaging on which the patterns dance around in a mesmerizing fashion in front of my eyes. There may be mirrors that confuse and trick my idea of distance and space. In amongst the blend of indistinguishable noises there may be someone who wants to talk to me. How can I possibly isolate the voice of one person in amongst the assortment of all the other sounds? The voice just merges into all the other sounds. There are so many things happening around, I cannot process all the data or stop my brain from trying to process it. In other words, I have no ability to concentrate on, or filter out, this constant bombardment of unreliable data from my senses. All I can do is use my logic to try and decipher the muddle. However, there is one advantage. I am much faster then the average person at scanning for a particular product on a shelf, providing I know exactly how the packaging looks. I quickly scan the shelf, then use my own pattern recognition strategy to determine which of the blurs is the most likely to be the required packet. (This scanning skill is also useful when looking for lost pins, butterfly backs for earrings, coins, etc on the floor.) I can only keep this up for a couple of seconds. Usually by the time I leave the shop my brain is in overdrive and worse still, my brain is likely to have already been in overdrive before I even reached the shop.

Shops are very tempting places. If I was left to my own devices and did not have to act in the 'normal' way, I would want to explore the shop, feeling, seeing, smelling, hearing what all the things are like! For instance, I like to put my hands into trays of small nails/screws and also find out what sounds I can produce from drinking glasses. But of course I know what all the do's and don'ts are in 'the world', so I without fail behave in the 'normal' way! The only way I can find consistency in 'the world' is to keep experiencing the way things are, until they make sense.

Any crowded situation causes me difficulties. I have never been keen on going to crowded places, which has always been a restricting factor in my social life. As a child I detested parties and made this quite clear to my mother. My parents decided that I must overcome my 'insecurities' and invariably made me go. However, my mother always made sure I was with a friend. As a child I thought that my parents were very heartless and uncaring about my feelings, which led me to believe that people do not have the same sort of emotions as myself. What would have happened to me if my mother had protected me from 'the world' and never made me go to school, shopping, parties? Even as an adult I find Parties, Discos, Pubs, Gatherings of people are very physically challenging environments. It would be so easy for me to say 'Going outside is too much of a hassle, I have had enough of compensating, from now on I will not even venture out of my bedroom', but this is not my way. In my life there is an inevitable trade off between doing activities that are exhausting and doing nothing. The art is to get the right balance.

There are many pitfalls for people like myself who perceive 'the world' via distorted senses. Given different circumstances my childhood confusions could so easily have lead to adult paranoia. There was a time when I nearly fell into the trap of becoming over anxious about hygiene. I was already in pain and tired so I wanted to ensure I did not become ill. At another time I wanted to keep the big bad outside world out of our home and started to become overly security conscious.

Some evidence once came to my attention, which suggested that people suffering from Dyslexia were more likely to have allergies and/or sensitivities to substances, compared with the 'normal' population[10]. Why?! As a child I suffered from eczema and now suffer from hay fever. To determine whether there is anything else which adversely affects me, I have had some allergy tests. These have indicated that there is a high possibility that I am allergic to things such as eggs, milk, cheese, chocolate, caffeine and many artificial colours and preservatives. Could I really be allergic to my staple diet?

To determine whether or not this is true, I have decided to simultaneously cut out of my diet for about 6 weeks, all the foods that it is suspected I am allergic or sensitive to. After several days of this 'new' diet I am feeling rather strange. It feels as if I am walking on air and as if the top section of my head is about half a metre above the rest of my head and body! (I had been eating properly, so these sensations were not due to a lack of food.) Could these strange feelings be withdrawal symptoms? It has also emerged that I am very sensitive to all sorts of chemicals released from e.g. paints, wallpaper pastes, varnishes, new carpet fumes, solvents, new plastics, new foams. If I avoid all the things, which I am sensitive to perhaps, I will feel healthier and will not constantly get terrible migraines. However, avoiding all the above chemicals and foods would not be very easy and could be very restricting. For instance, if I worked in an office and it was completely refurbished I would not be able to go to work for months, maybe years!

After several weeks, I have noticed that I feel generally more healthy. I no longer have a headache after eating a meal and my energy level is much more even throughout the day. I used to be in a terrible state for about an hour before dinner, wandering around in a daze and unable to think about anything other than my desperate hunger; it was a craving for food. I would often eat biscuits, but they did not appease my appetite for more substantial food. It never occurred to me that this behaviour was odd. Up until now my family had just accepted, without comment, that this was my way of functioning. Now, I no longer have the awful lows in my energy level, but I miss the highs! I think this explains my childhood craving to lick all the sticky from 'sticky-backed' envelopes/paper and to eat mint flavoured toothpaste.

Some of the things I am sensitive to can give me enormous highs and it feels as if every nerve ending around my whole body is alive and tingling. The tingling can be overwhelming and the only way to alleviate it is to keep on the move. When I am like this I feel as if I could run a marathon. Often after being exposed to such chemicals and as the 'high' wears off, I feel as if I have the flu with a migraine. If I am to stay feeling healthy in the future I will need to avoid all the things I am allergic/sensitive too.

My perception of taste is in some way inconstant. I do not notice the subtle differences in flavour of foods. For instance, I can taste the difference between a potato and carrot, but am unable to appreciate that different varieties of potato have distinctive flavours. I find it hard to determine whether the food I am eating has the

---

[10] I believe this is also true of those suffering from ADD, Dyspraxia and Autism.

correct taste. This confusion in my sense of taste causes me a basic problem, which is I am unlikely to taste the subtle change in flavour of a piece of food which is going bad. Is my sense of taste impaired? Or is my memory of how things taste, poor? How does my sense of smell fit into the picture? I seem unable to find the consistency. Sometimes I eat a piece of food and to me it tastes like a completely different food or substance. For example potato may taste like carrot! Or a tomato may taste the same as oil paint!? Often when confronted by food, for my own peace of mind, I ask the people around me whether it tastes alright, to be sure that it is not poisonous! For me, eating is just a necessity of life. Most people find it strange that I receive no pleasure from eating, but they do not understand that taste is just one more thing that bombards my confused senses.

Everybody has terrible trouble comprehending my disability, so I have written a report about the differences between the way my body behaves relative to the 'normal' person, so that my friends and relations can have a better idea of my physical perceptions[11] e.g. sight, hearing, etc. The report is written in a stark and logical style listing my physical problems. It reads more like a science textbook than a novel! This has caused one fundamental problem. Unless the person reading it is very interested in the exact details of my problems, it is very boring! However, those of my family and friends who have read the report seem to have a much better idea of 'my world', although they often find it difficult to imagine. The understanding that they have gained from my report has resulted in them becoming much more tolerant towards me. For the first time, my parents seem to have a fairly good idea of whom I am and this has improved their attitude towards me.

As I typed the report (typing is easier than writing), my poor English was a real problem. My mother took on the arduous job of turning my words into meaningful sentences and paragraphs. Despite my effort, in every line there were at least three or four grammatical errors and many spelling mistakes. The word processing package on my computer was able to correct some of the spellings, using the 'spell checking' facility, but unfortunately many of my words were so badly spelt that the 'spell checker' was unable to find the correct word! Perhaps I need a computer with a microphone that would allow me to dictate my work, as this would save time and effort with respect to both typing and spelling.

The computer I use has a cathode-ray tube (CRT) type of screen as opposed to the Liquid Crystal Display (LCD) screen of a notebook computer. This CRT screen is very hard on my eyes and if I spend any length of time looking at it my eyesight rapidly deteriorates. I am told this is often a problem for people suffering from 'Scotopic Sensitivity Syndrome' because the CRT screens flicker. Ideally I need a notebook computer with the LCD screen, since they do not flicker[12].

---

[11] At this time my thinking had not gone far enough for me to grasp the connections between my physical state and my psychological reactions, thus the report did not deal with any psychology or my perceptions of people.

[12] I could not have written this book without my notebook computer and its LCD screen.

I find it frustrating and annoying that anything I express in English is only an approximation of what I really mean. I have equal difficulty conveying my thoughts in both written and verbal form. Very often I am unsure which words to use and unable to find the right combination of words. Often my approximations are not really close enough to what I really mean to project. I can translate words back into my wordless mind much easier than I can turn my wordless thoughts into meaningful articulate, accurate words. Words are only a human devised way of communication and are not an evolutionary trait, so is this disruption in my language caused because I have had limited exposure to language due to my sight and hearing problems? Or do I have an inherent language disability?

To make matters worse I often have great difficulty recalling words. This often results in me saying or writing something that is a very poor approximation of what I mean. A trivial example could be that I may wish to say 'My books are under the shelf', but I may get halfway through the sentence and be unable to recall the word 'under' and then end up saying 'My books are not on the shelf'. (Whilst writing this book much time was spent choosing the correct words.)

Writing the report about my disabilities made me realise that I can not continue hating all the people who have tormented me. There was no way they could have known what they were doing to me. How could the teachers who laughed at my inability to read, have known that my vision was different? How could my parents have known that I could not walk properly because I had poor balance? How could my sister have known that playing music while I was studying was genuinely disrupting my concentration? How could my friends have known that I could not discern left from right because my brain worked differently? How could my friend's mother have known that the reason I could not pronounce the word 'hospital' was because I could not distinguish the individual sounds which made up the word? How could anyone have known that when placing a teacup on a table I needed to listen out for it hitting the table, so that I knew when to let go of it - banging things down was due to a lack of distance awareness, not anger. There is an endless list of people who never had a chance of comprehending my environment. I must reach the point where I can forgive all the people who misunderstood me, for the only person being harmed by the hate is me.

I will always have the problem that people I meet, who never get to know me well, will never understand me. This causes me to feel a certain amount of isolation. For me this is just one of the hazards of living. However, I find it very irritating when people in a position to understand me, are simply too narrow-minded to comprehend 'my world' and insist on continually blundering on in ignorance. Can the minds of such people be opened or are they a lost cause?

Now that I understand my environment, is it now time for me to return to university? My compensations are so extremely complex and finely balanced that they make the concepts that I have learnt from college and my short time at university, seem extremely easy and uncomplicated. I have refined and whittled down my strategies to the bare minimum, so that there is more room in my mind for studying. There is one thing which really scares me; the pain. For the most part I can think the pain away, but if the pain becomes too severe there is nothing that I can do about it. The greatest problem is, the more I do the more pain I am in. Within me there is still a burning desire for knowledge and I see no other way of fulfilling it, other than to return to university and restart the first year of the Honours Degree in Electronics. A friend posed the question,

"What have you got to lose by returning to university?" I feel the answer is 'nothing'. I will not have lost anything if I return to university and find that I am still unable to cope, it could not be any worse than wondering for the rest of my life whether I could have completed the course. Will my new found knowledge of my environment be enough to enable me to complete even one year at university?

2

....Re-starting the honours degree course in Electronic Engineering at university. The university found me a quieter room in the top corner of a student accommodation block. For most of this academic year I was aged 23....

I know exactly what to expect here at university, I now have ways of dealing with the barrage of stimuli, which bombard my distorted muddled senses. To complete the academic year I will have to endure much pain and tiredness, I will fight them with all the logic that I can muster and strive to shut myself off from the reality of the pain. I must endeavour to control my emotional responses and think in a calm and logical way. This will be necessary for my sanity, because I am effectively torturing myself by making my body do all the required academic work. It is very hard doing activities day after day, which I know, will be extremely painful. My new understanding of the extent of my physical problems enables me to cope with my physical limitations and to better judge my boundaries. This understanding has given me a feeling of calm acceptance, which has in turn reduced my frustration.

Here at university, nobody understands very much about my disability and because it is so complex, it is impossible to educate anyone about myself in a few sentences. There is a sense in which this no longer worries me. Even if someone did fully comprehend, they could not take away the pain or the tiredness. Besides, I have coped for most of my life surrounded by people who did not understand me, so one more year will not hurt. I am accustomed to being self-reliant and no longer hate myself, therefore being alone, although not ideal, is not really a problem.

My main concern is creating the right balance between work and rest. Maybe if I can achieve this, my life will not be too unbearable. Each day I do as little academic work as possible, which involves going to the lectures and doing the work sheets of related exercises. To gain understanding of a new concept, I work through specific examples. For me, this is easier than reading through lots of words which are explaining the concept. My work schedule is organised so that I work for about twenty minutes and then rest for as long as necessary in order to recuperate. I spend more time resting, than I do working owing to the tiredness and pain.

The textbooks decorate the bookshelf and are only ever read on the rare occasions when I have not understood something, even then I only read selected paragraphs, never whole chapters or complete books. This worries me because the lecturers are always advising plenty of background reading. My lack of reading is not due to laziness or because I cannot read, it is simply too hard on my eyes. Although I do have a problem in that my reading age is equivalent to that a twelve and a half year old, the technical words are not a problem. It is just some of the adjoining descriptive words which I have trouble with. When reading I have no perception of phrasing, emphasis or punctuation. (Having little idea about punctuation makes writing reports very tough.) Reading soon becomes very boring since I am unable to read any faster than normal speaking speed and the more I read, the slower it becomes. Strangely, my spelling age is equivalent to that of a thirteen year old, does this mean I can spell more words than I can read?!

I find concepts easy to understand and manipulate, but have difficulty understanding the words used to describe them. Fortunately at this level, in Electronics many mathematical equations, circuit diagrams and graphs are used to describe ideas and these are easier for me to comprehend, because they are logical. After all, logic is my foundation for finding consistency.

My insight into Physics and Mathematical equations helps me to fill in the gaps between what I perceive and what is actually happening in 'the world'. For instance, I often feel as if I could just fall off the face of the earth into space, but knowledge of gravity persuades me that this will definitely not happen! My logical analysis of 'the world' does not give me a sense of security, but rather a framework of understanding. However, this does not remove the underlying feelings of insecurity caused by my senses deceiving me; given the same circumstances anyone would suffer these fears. I still feel as frightened as I did in my childhood, but the difference now is that I can overlay logic on top of my fears, which gives me a sense of 'logical' security. This enables me to block out or deal with any underlying feelings of fear. My knowledge about 'my world' compared to 'the world' also helps me to understand the way I feel. In some ways I no longer need to be overly concerned with trying to be a perfectionist at behaving 'normally'. I now accept myself much more for who I really am.

To overcome my problem of time disorientation I have a digital watch with an alarm and an Electronic Personal Organiser. Each week I type in the next week's schedule and set the alarms so that they ring when I should be going somewhere. This device has taken an enormous weight off my mind and I no longer worry about when it will be time to go somewhere. One of the most time consuming weekly activities is the practical laboratory work. I find it very tiring making up circuit boards and taking measurements, these things require plenty of fine muscle control over my hands and eyes. I understand that this is a price that I have to pay.

Ever since I began to comprehend the details of my physical difficulties, there has been this recurring question going through my mind, a day does not pass without me asking it; What is the purpose of human existence? I live in so much pain and everything takes so much effort that for me there needs to be a reason to carry on living. One day whilst having a shower, I had a flash of inspiration; everyone, no matter what their circumstances, has the potential to make the most of everything they have within their own situation, without exploitation. Is this the whole answer or part of the answer to my question? What are my assets? What should I be making the most of?

Another question that is plaguing my mind is; are the objects called people, important? Do people have any relevance to me? Maybe, if I could become 'normal' I could become a 'real' person and then people would be relevant because I would be on equal terms. I would dearly love to become a 'real' person and be able to have the chance to interact with people. But how do I become a 'real' person? Perhaps one day I will be able to get rid of the ghosts of people within my mind and have 'real live human' friends whom understand me? The only real live friends I have do not understand me and I have to interact with them on their level which is rather one sided. Why are people such a mystery to me?

It is a great shame that I cannot use my spare time to join in some of the many activities on the university campus, if I had this opportunity I might discover more about 'people'. Extracurricular activities would be a huge drain on my energy level. Before returning to university, I knew that the only way for me to have enough energy to pass the course, was to sacrifice any potential social life. It is tragic coming to a place where there are so many opportunities and being unable to take advantage of them. I greatly regret and am frustrated by the restrictions on my extracurricular activities. To my great sorrow my so-called 'social life' is confined to chatting with the people on my course and those who live nearby in the student accommodation.

On the odd occasion when I have enough energy to walk around part of the campus, I will carry my camera with me and take some wildlife photographs, mainly of the resident ducks and geese! This gives me a sense of achievement and for a short time gives me something creative to do. During late autumn and early winter, when the sun rises over the horizon between about seven and eight o'clock, from the vantage point on the 3rd floor close to my bedroom, I managed to take some sunrise pictures. Many people seem to think that much of my photography is very good and are surprised that I have never been taught in any form, especially considering my visual problems. Somehow I just know what to do. I tend to take close-ups of particular objects such as toadstools or leaves, but I would never be able to photograph the objects called people because I do not understand them. Once an object or sky scene has been frozen in time on a photograph, I can then try to understand more about it. Often it is easier for me to see something on a photograph because there are less visual distortions (outside light causes more distortions than inside 'natural' bulb lighting).

It is a struggle for me to do everyday things, such as see, hear, walk etc. that I am aware that it makes me more vulnerable to outside stresses and pressures (getting work done on time). After all, there is only so much that anyone can take. It is not only the academic work that puts a great demand on my resources, particularly my energy. There are all the other things that need to be done such as washing clothes, small amounts of shopping, etc. Even such things as going to the canteen to eat a meal, having a shower, walking to lectures etc. all cause drains on my energy level. My whole life revolves around discerning between what is necessity and what is merely 'a nicety'.

With all the compromises that I have made to both my extracurricular and academic life, I am managing to keep more-or-less on top of the workload. But as the year progresses I am becoming increasingly tired. Having completed two terms, my energy level has become very low. All I can do in the holiday period is rest. Once the holiday has finished there will be seven weeks before the end of year exams. This will be my make or break time. I intend to spend the six weeks before the exams going through all the notes I made during lectures and make very compact revision notes. I never rewrote any of my lecture notes or even re-read them because my eyes were too painful. Going through all my notes is a mammoth job and one that seems never-ending.

As the exam week draws near, my revision is just about on schedule, but the exhaustion is becoming overwhelming. In order to continue studying I have focused on the task in hand, to the total exclusion of everything else going on around me. This is a defensive strategy. At this stage I must not be disturbed by the pain or tiredness and the only way is not to look forward or backwards and to block out my physical reality. I know that I can not keep this up for very long, but there are only a few weeks until the exams will be over.

I am now truly exhausted from reading all my lecture notes. Having condensed the lecture notes into concise crib notes I rely solely on reading the crib notes before each exam. It is now very hard for me to control myself and stay focused, because the pain is overwhelming, but so far I am beating it. How will I fare in the exams when I am relying solely on my notes taken during lectures, rather than complementing my knowledge with background reading? I will need to use all my last reserves of energy and tenacity to complete the exams. The university agreed that I should be allowed to write my answers on blue coloured paper (It is easier for me to see writing on such paper because it reduces some of my visual distortions). They also agreed to print the exam papers on blue, and that I should have some extra time in the exams because of the severity of my Dyslexia.

After completing all but the last exam we have a weekend break. The final exam to be taken is mathematics. This is my weakest subject, purely because I have not had enough time to fill in all the gaps in my knowledge. I arrived at university at a gross disadvantage because I do not have an 'A' level in mathematics, the mathematics I did at HNC level while at college was very narrow. I know how to temporarily restore my energy supplies so that I can do some decent revision. All I need is a packet of 'peppermint' sweets! Years ago when I was at work I used to supplement my energy supplies by eating peppermint sweets. For some reason peppermint sweets give me huge bursts of energy. I become hyperactive. It feels as if my whole body has an electrified life force within it. I have always used them to enable me to get through low energy days in my life. But now at university I will need to eat them for the whole weekend and all of Monday. This seems the only way for me to find a way through the exhaustion. What effects will eating mints for so many days have on me?

It worked, the peppermint sweets enabled me to have just enough energy to finish my revision and do the mathematics exam. The week of the exams has been one of the most difficult of my life. I can relax now because there is nothing else which desperately needs to be done this academic year. The relief is enormous. I can now rest. This year at university has given me a great sense of being part of 'the world'. Normally I feel as if I live purely in 'my world', but on an academic technical level I have been able to effectively communicate with people.

Finally the last day of term has come and I will find out my results of the exams and assignments. My average mark was 79%, which puts me on line for a 'first'. My marks varied greatly from 50% to 100%! 50% for a computing assignment, where I misinterpreted what I see as slippery ambiguous words written by the lecturer to describe the aim of the assignment! 100% for an end of year exam. Mostly my marks were between the mid 60%'s to the mid 80%'s. At last I know without a shadow of a doubt that I am definitely not stupid, it is like a huge weight has been lifted off my mind. Despite being very tired I cannot wait to go home and have a rest and then to return here next year to do the second year of the course.

Having been home for two weeks it is becoming obvious that I am physically exhausted and mentally drained. Understandably the company who sponsored me through the academic year at university, wishes me to go and work for them during the summer holidays. I have agreed to do 6 weeks work and then rest for the remaining 6 weeks before the start of the university term. It is torturous going back to work in this drained state and working in an unfamiliar department with people who are unknown to me. Every day seems to last for an eternity and although I do not have a huge amount of work to do it is still further depleting my energy supplies.

There is one benefit from working, earning money. This has enabled me to buy a new musical instrument; an Electronic Keyboard. Many years ago I tried and failed to learn to play the piano, because my sight was not good enough to read the music and my control over my fingers was too poor. However, now I have better control over my fingers and intend only to read the tune off a piece of music and then improvise the whole accompaniment, using the guitar chords written on the music as a guide to how it should sound. (After 9 months I had become proficient enough to be asked to play the piano for a local 'special' church service on a weekday. I accepted the challenge and nervously accompanied a large group of singing elderly ladies!! At the time of writing this book I had reached a level of about Grade 7/8.)

After being at home for about 10 weeks it is quite obvious that my energy supplies are not going to recover in time to start back at university. My energy level is just too depleted. This is a heartbreaking and depressing setback; sometimes life seems so unjust. It is so frustrating to think that I will have to wait a whole year before returning to my course. I can not believe it, after all this time my life is still hampered by my disability. I can compensate fairly well for the physical disability but not for the secondary effects of tiredness and pain, although I am told I have an extremely high pain threshold. If I had never learnt to compensate for my disability my body would not become tired or painful, but without these strategies there would be no way for me to have done so many things such as going to university. There is no easy answer to the question; How much should an individual compensate?

3

....Year away from university spent at home resting and recuperating. For most of this academic year I was aged 24....

People, including my parents, expect me to understand how they are feeling, but I have no idea how to interpret or comprehend their emotions. The emotions of other people are a mystery to me. Throughout my life this has been a huge problem and has often caused me to inadvertently behave in an inappropriate fashion, resulting in other people becoming upset or very cross. This produces tremendous problems in my interactions with people at home and in all areas of my life. When I was a young child this did not really matter, but the older I became the more people expected of me.

I have found it hard to grasp the social code by which my parents expect me to live. Often their rules seemed either meaningless or contradictory. In many ways people are not my first priority, they are too complex and different from myself. People are 'objects' which are just part of 'the world'. Is there anyone else like me in 'the world'? My first priorities relate to my own survival and making some consistent sense of 'the world' in which I and 'my world' regretfully exist.

During my life, my parents have drummed into me a code of conduct, which gives me guidelines on acceptable social behaviour and I have learnt how to behave in a polite fashion (in most circumstances!). Thankfully, my parents managed to restrain my 'disrespect' for 'everything'. It could have easily led me to criminal activities. On the whole I can deal with people in passing, but do not know how to interact on a more familiar level, because they expect me to be able to understand their behaviour. It is hard enough trying to interpret people from their verbal communications without trying to understand their body language. For instance, just by looking at a person I cannot tell if they are feeling unwell or tired. Since people do not realise my inability to understand them, it is preferable to keep everyone at arms length and guessing at what I might do next.

At eighteen years old I started studying the characters in television soap operas and have now learnt the raw basics of behaviour. I have deduced that different situations make 'normal' people react in particular ways and even more confusing, the same situation can make different people react in dissimilar ways. It is hard to deduce why certain people behave in certain ways and impossible to anticipate who will react in which manner. The way other people react to even the simplest situations is often different from the way I would react. This is why I use logic to enable me to act in a reasonable way. My reactions are based on reasoned past observation and experience. For instance, whilst watching a film recently, one scene made my sister suddenly cringe. It would never have occurred to me that this specific scene was gruesome or worth cringing about. (My sister reacts to things in a fairly 'standard' fashion.) If I were to watch the film again or saw a similar scene in another film, I would know that it was gruesome and would probably pretend to cringe!

It is a mystery to me the way people interact with each other on a familiar level. It is an even bigger mystery as to why they use 'touch' when it obviously causes an overwhelming number of confusing sensations. My skin is so sensitive that I can feel gnats if they land on me (I can brush them away before I get bitten). Why does a mother put her arms around her crying child? Or, why does a person put their arms around a friend who is upset? What is the purpose of touch? Where is the consistency? I am confused.

I only grasp the extreme emotions (e.g. ecstatically happy, livid), I have these emotions, but somehow there is an inconsistency. Relating to the nuances of human behaviour seems impossible. On the whole, nobody ever treats me as if they comprehend even my extreme feelings, let alone any other responses. This leaves me without any motivation to understand theirs. To me 'the world' seems a stony hard and uncaring place. Are my emotional responses completely different from those of other people?

From the time I was last at university, I have wondered whether people are important. The idea that people might be important came to me after an acquaintance was tragically killed in a car crash. All his friends were horrified and have been grief-stricken since the accident, about 6 months ago. This accident also brought into focus in my mind the sheer fragility of life on this planet. There are so many things that could kill any of us at any given time. This in turn raises the question, is there a purpose to life, a reason for living? I am going to try and discover more about people on a personal level, in order to try and deduce whether people and/or life are important.

Up until now, communicating with anyone has been like shouting across a crowded noisy room, to someone standing on the other side. The person on the other side can hear very little of what I am saying, equally I can hear only fragments of what they are saying. Neither of us can hear enough of each other to make any real sense of what is being said. Looking back on my life, I can think of several people who have tried really hard to reach me, but the gulf between 'my world' and 'the world' has been too wide. Somehow I must find a way of walking across that imaginary noisy crowded room, so that I can communicate with someone, but whom should I try and communicate with?

Shortly before I went to university, I wrote a report listing all my physical problems. I have thrown this report across to the other side of the imaginary crowded room, in the hope that someone who reads it will be able to understand something about me and then actually reach me.

Recently, I have been helping an untutored pianist to gain enough confidence to be able to play in church services. This has meant that we needed to spend several hours together each week, practising (I play flute). During this time we have obviously been talking and this pianist is trying to reach me, trying to find out how I perceive. My use of the English Language is improving all the time and is reaching the point where I can have a fairly reasonable attempt at communicating my perceptions. I am still shouting across my imaginary crowded room but the pianist is beginning to understand much of what I am saying. At last someone is hearing me. This is exciting but also frightening, supposing this person expects me to understand or trust them! Do I really want to let anyone into 'my world'?

During the coming months we were to both start walking across the imaginary room towards each other. The closer we got the less we had to shout and the more we heard, the more we understood of each other and with time we met in the middle. I can now see that the pianist is a person and this person has come to understand a huge amount about my environment. This person has become a friend, Valerie. Never before has anyone come so close to understanding 'my world' and neither have I ever had such easy access to the ways of 'the world'. This friendship has created a life changing flow of understanding between 'my world' and 'the world'.

I have spent many hours talking to Valerie about the emotional traumatic events in her life. This has been a great revelation. Now for the first time in my life I have come to realise that other people feel things in much the same way as myself. The only differences between Valerie and myself are the circumstances, not the emotional responses. Emotionally I am no different from anyone else because my emotional responses are relevant to my physical environment. My perception of 'the world' is unreliable and faulty and therefore 'my world' is a confusing and physically hostile place in which to live. For instance if a 'normal' person is at the receiving end of some hostile abuse, they in some way feel frightened, equally I feel frightened in 'my world'. An example of this would be if I walk through a room full of noisy people I feel frightened, because I cannot make proper sense of what is happening around me; my fear is justified. It is only by appreciating my physical environment that it is possible to empathise with my behaviour, fear and despair.

After many more hours of talking with Valerie, it became crystal clear that there was nothing odd about my reactions. After all, how well would someone from 'the world' mentally cope if we swapped bodies?! How well would they cope with sight and hearing distortions, faulty balance, poor co-ordination and the isolation of being totally misunderstood? Valerie has now become my interface and forms a link between my lack of awareness of peoples' emotions and 'the world' of 'normal' interaction. Now with this link between where I am and 'the world' of interaction I am able to learn about and understand people much better. At last I am making some consistent sense. Now maybe, one day I may reach the point where the nuances of other peoples' emotions make consistent sense. Will I ever be able to gauge how other people are feeling? If I could make real sense of people, my computer may no longer be my best friend.

It has been up to me to teach my parents, family and friends how I perceive, so that they have the opportunity to grasp my situation. This learning has been mutual because in my quest for truth I have now come a very long way to understanding people in 'the world'. The silhouettes and ghosts of people, who understood me and lived only within the confines of my mind, have been banished. They are now superfluous because my parents and Valerie have a reasonable understanding of me. I think removing the 'ghosts' is another step I have taken along the road to normality.

Throughout my life people have frequently let me down because they did not know my perspective of 'life'. Equally my body is always failing me, because it sends me faulty information about my surroundings. It is therefore hardly surprising that I have trouble trusting anyone or anything. I use logic and probability estimation to replace 'normal' trust. For instance, if I am walking on the pavement and I hear a car travelling along the road, I know that it is very improbable that the car will hit me, providing I remain on the pavement. Another example is, if I am going to sit on my bedroom chair, I deduce that the chair has never collapsed before, therefore it is unlikely to break when I sit down this time. Now that I understand what trust is and my reasons for not having any, will I ever be able to attain 'real' trust? Or can 'real' trust only be based on stability? Stability is not part of 'my world' of inconsistency. Maybe one day I will be able to trust people?

I have always had tremendous trouble projecting my feelings. Expressing myself in words has been very difficult. It has been so hard to make consistent sense that I have needed to spend years working out how to project my feelings effectively. For instance, if I am angry or think that I should feel angry, I might wish to act in an angry way. From experience I know that cross people slam things, clench their fists, frown, shout or growl. So if I wish to appear cross I do these things to back up my words. It is no good using angry words without the appropriate voice and body language. Equally it would be unconvincing to smile whilst saying 'I am very depressed' or to say in an expressionless voice 'I am very happy'. I started creating appropriate facial expressions and a few gestures while I was still at junior school and then progressed on to hand gestures and more advanced body language during my years at work. Working out how to project myself has never struck me as strange, until recently, when I discovered that to most people it comes naturally!

Getting my voice to make the correct tone is hard and even now after all these years, I still slip up. Sometimes I may forget and use a tone at random and as a result am completely misinterpreted. Consequently, when I speak I must always remember to act in an appropriate way. Similarly, if someone is speaking to me it is necessary to act in an appropriate manner. For instance, if someone is angry I must endeavour not to laugh! Equally if someone is upset I must not smile, or if someone is happy I must not look completely blank. It is even harder trying to react to the nuances of another's behaviour. I now fully realise that the majority of people react to others depending on exactly how they are treated. People spark off each other and it is true to say that every action causes a reaction. All these aspects of human interaction have taken me years to master but they still do not come naturally.

Being back at home this year is having its compensations. I have time to do things such as playing the flute and electronic keyboard, drawing, photography. But most satisfying is my new found insights into 'people'. In a sense I have time to find myself. In one way this can be dangerous, because I do not always like what I find, but on the other hand it is necessary for me to try to make consistent sense of 'the world' and my place in it. These things do not really make up for the lack of intellectual stimulation at home. I miss the stimulation of the course and 'very clever' people at university.

On the whole I now cope fairly well with most things. There is nothing I will not do providing there is a good reason. For example, I would not go for a drive in a car just for the sake of it, why should I give myself a headache for no reason? However, if I decided I needed to go somewhere, provided someone could drive me, I would just get in the car and go! Throughout my whole life I have tried to discern between necessary and unnecessary things in order to keep my pain and disorientation within reasonable bounds.

Until now I have never had to deal with moving house! My family last moved house when I was about one and a half years old. (I can actually remember moving and even our previous home!) My home is my reference point and has been my stable, unchanging sanctuary for most of my life. Complete terror strikes my heart every time my parents even mention the words 'moving house'. It now seems inevitable that my family will move to a bigger house in the same village, so that the four of us are not so cramped. The thought of moving house is petrifying. I can think of nothing more destabilising than to be removed from my prime place of safety and my main reference point, my home. It is hard to make my parents understand how much of a critical and fundamental reference point the house is. They perceive my resistance to moving as a passing phase and something I will easily become used to after a few days. When I have been to university, or away from home, I could, at any time if desired, return to my reference point, at home.

The reason for the house being a fundamental reference point is that I do not have my own internal security. This means that I do not feel safe within my own body/environment because of my faulty, inconsistent perceptions of 'the world' (e.g. poor sight, hearing, balance etc.). These feelings of insecurity would have swallowed me up and made me mentally ill if I had been unable to create my own reference system. This means that instead of having my own internal natural references for security like 'normal' people, I have created external reference systems. Changing my external reference system to another house will be torturous. I do not think that I would have made it through life if my family had kept moving house. In fact I come from an extremely stable background. My parents did not split up, we never moved house, we lived in a village in a cul-de-sac at the edge of fields, my father was always employed, and nothing traumatic ever happened to the family. This stability has been the making of me and has enabled me to create good strong external reference systems.

The day has come, the one that I have been dreading for most of my life. It is today that we must move house. I am spending the whole day at Valerie's home, a place that I know well. This place is now my only tenuous reference point in the whole world. I feel awash, alone, empty and unstable without my home as a reference. Nobody really understands, even Valerie is struggling.

The days, weeks and months have passed. Maybe one day our 'new' house will seem like home, but not yet. The small home of Valerie has become my prime reference point and in the meantime I am trying to create a sensible set of parameters and references in the new house. Much decorating is being done at the new house, which is adding to my problems, because I am allergic to so many glues, pastes and paints. I cope with my allergies by staying away from the things that are a problem. This means I am spending much time away from the 'new' home. At times these allergies and sensitivities put irritating restrictions on my life.

I do not always perceive 'the world' in the same way. I have different modes of thinking. For instance, sometimes I perceive the head of a human as a purely information receiving and processing centre. The eyes as processing light, the ears processing sound and the nose processing smell. Alternatively, I look at a ball and think of it only in terms of what sound it makes when it hits different surfaces. Or I may look at a yacht on the sea and consider it only in terms of density. The low density air pushes the high density yacht through the medium density sea. By this I mean, to me, the yacht which is solid (i.e. high density), is being pushed through the sea (medium density), by the wind (low density). In other words I perceive the picture of a yacht on the sea, not as a pure object but in terms of physical forces, density and movement. These ways of 'mono' thinking are very powerful in finding consistency and have been a huge help to me in determining what 'the world' is like. This type of very clear thinking is deep within me and far beyond the world of slippery, inconsistent, inadequate language.

When I was a child, my parents very often had terrible trouble communicating with me and particularly explaining things to me because I was very often thinking in completely different terms to them. Sometimes my parents realised this and would start explaining things from different angles, but mostly my way of thinking was (and often still is) so foreign, that they never managed to reach me. It has been up to me to build the interface between 'my world' and 'the world' to enable me to reach out to where 'normal' people are. My compensations and strategies are like bridges between worlds.

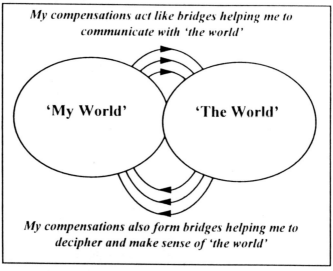

* What happens if the worlds are too far part?
* How would people know to say 'I see differently', 'I hear differently', etc if they have never experienced anything other than their own environment?
* How difficult is it to understand a world different from your own?
* What happens to less intelligent people with problems similar to mine? Do they get classed as mentally handicapped when paradoxically they are not of low intelligence, but are simply unable to build the bridges to the world?
* If a person is genuinely mentally handicapped, what chance have they got of managing to build bridges?
* Do people get classified as mentally ill when in fact they are dealing with their very different physical environment in a way which is relevant to 'their world'?

EIGHT

Moving Out Into The World

1

....September 1994. Academic year spent at home. I have swallowed my pride and am returning to 'my old college' which in my absence has become a university! I am studying mathematics one morning a week. (By June 1995 I had attained distinctions in all the subjects with an average mark of about 91%). Having been at a very good university in a well run department, returning to 'my old college' came as a bit of a culture shock. I knew that it would frustrate and irritate me if I had to study at 'my old college' on a full time basis, as it would not be very academically challenging. Ideally I need to find some way back to my university degree course. I am now a quarter of a century old and I want to define the nature of my problems in terms that everybody can understand....

Many years ago, Edna suggested that perhaps I could teach people suffering from Dyslexia, to read and write, as I would be able to empathise with them. But, what is my disability? Do my problems fit neatly into the known sections of medical science? What can be learnt about my problems, which will help other people who have similar difficulties? I need to consider exactly how my problems can be defined, by using terminology that anyone can grasp. I am intrigued by such questions as, what is Dyslexia and do anomalies in the development of reflexes have any relevance to Dyslexia? Why does my brain work differently? What aspect of my brain is different? Is it chemical? Is it physical? A mixture of both?

Various professionals appearing to make uninformed diagnoses have heightened my curiosity into the exact nature of my condition:-

- (mid 1970's to mid 1980's) Endless teachers seemed to think that my Dyslexia was purely due to one or more of the following: stupidity, laziness, carelessness, a wish not to learn, my upbringing, a fussy mother!

- (late 1980's) An ophthalmologist appeared to say there could not be anything wrong with my vision, because Dyslexia is a purely psychological problem and that her neurologist friends agreed with her!

- (late 1980's) I was advised to become relaxed at all times, but I ignored the advice, claiming that it was ludicrous for me to completely remove all of my compensations and relax, because I would be totally lost in the chaos. Now years later, many professional people agree with me and they also believe the removal of my compensations would have caused me to become unreachable.

- (early 1990's) A perplexed neurologist appeared to imply that I was suffering from M.E. and thought I should attend an M.E. clinic, but appeared to back down when I pointed out that the medical evidence did not support this theory!

- (mid 1990's) During a consultation a neurologist appeared to continually try to put his words into my mouth and as far as I understand openly said that he did not believe I had distortions in my sight, hearing etc. He appeared to believe that I definitely needed behavioural therapy. I tried to explain that altering my behaviour and compensations without taking account of my physical problems was a terrible idea (most people agree with me), but he did not seem to agree! Following the three hour consultation he wrote what I can only describe as a twisted report, using what I believe were his assumptions and words. The report bears little relevance to my case! Throughout the consultation and in the subsequent report, it appears that he felt my condition was purely psychological! I have subsequently discovered that, as yet, there are no neurological tests that can prove that someone like myself has distortions in their sight, hearing etc. I know there are many cases of people who have been misdiagnosed as having psychological, neurotic and/or behavioural disorders when the true underlying problem is with the physical make up of the brain.

My teachers and doctors should have been discovering which came first, the physiological or the psychological - but I believe they lacked the relevant information. They needed to have the knowledge to ask and discover the answers to questions such as; Is Alison's slow educational development affected by any one or a combination of low intelligence, disrupted childhood, social deprivation or faulty neurology? Can Alison not learn to read because of faulty vision? Does balance affect Alison's performance in Sports and deter her from going to crowded places? Exactly what is Alison perceiving? etc., etc........

Unfortunately, in my experience, educationalists, teachers, researchers, doctors and psychologists are too often busily working in their own little area. This meant that occasionally someone would recognise a very small part of my difficulties but they could not take stock of the wider picture (i.e. see me as a whole person).

Many people have asked me,

"Why didn't you tell someone you could not see, hear, taste, etc. properly?" The answer is simple. How could I possibly have known the differences in the way that I perceive, when the only experience I had of life was looking at the world through my own distorted senses. I had no frame of reference by which to answer such a question. For example, as a child, I never said, 'I cannot read because I cannot see' since I was unaware that my vision was different. How could I possibly have known what 'normal' people see. It took me a long time and many very detailed conversations with my immediate family to discover what my differences were. I am sure that most people with problems like mine never make the conceptual jump between 'their world' and 'the world'. I know people are unable to make the conceptual jump between their 'normal world' and 'my world'.

My way of operating is not wrong, but different, since it relates to my different physical environment and my way of compensating bridges the gap between 'my world' and 'the world'. My compensations are physiological and psychological devices for coping and are a vital part of my survival. The interplay between them is extremely complex. I am constantly searching for more efficient ways of compensating. The main difficulty is that there is always a trade off between the disability and the effort used in compensation. Firstly, if I under-compensated, my life would be unacceptably restricted e.g. without adequate compensation for my balance problems I would be unable to step outside of my home. Secondly, if I overcompensated I would always be unacceptably tired e.g. if I always used the huge exhausting compensation I use for crowded places. Therefore, I have created compensations that I can temporarily extend to allow me to do a more challenging task, or temporarily retract when they are not required.

Compensation comes at a price. Firstly mental fatigue is the result of the extensive conscious effort required and secondly, tired and aching muscles result from extensive muscle control over particular parts of my body e.g. my hand and arm when writing.

'Practise makes perfect', is this really true? In my experience, 'practise' is necessary to improve and can help in the development of compensations, but 'perfect' cannot be reached if there is a physical disability in the way. For example, it is obvious that I will never be able to speed read while I can only simultaneously see a few letters of ordinary written text!

For me, being open to all possibilities is an essential part of life and I believe that arrogance and professional pride are no excuse for ignorance. I would like all people to understand that not everyone perceives 'the world' in the same way. So exactly how have I made sense of what is going on?

The first thing I realised was that Dyslexia, Dyspraxia, ADD (& ADHD), and Autism have their own main characteristics which makes them distinct from each other, these are very briefly, as follows:-

- *The main characteristic of Dyslexia, is the inability to recognise words on a page and simultaneously translate them into something of meaning. This results in problems with reading and this naturally has the effect of causing poor spelling and grammar. It is impossible for me to recognise words because I do not see more than a few letters at any one time. If I could see whole words would I recognise them? As a young child I could not consistently recognise even two or three letter words. So am I Dyslexic? The special teaching directed at sufferers of Dyslexia instructs us on how to compensate for our problem(s). Surely it is not curing the underlying physical problems? Teaching me to read obviously does not alter my vision!! According to an official assessment, I am Dyslexic. Is Dyslexia the outward result of something much deeper?*

- *To an extent I am like many Dyspraxic sufferers, in that I have problems with clumsiness, co-ordination and can be sluggish in some physical movements as a result of poor fine and gross muscle control. However, I am not as badly affected* as most people who are classified as Dyspraxic. Consequently, physical activities such as sports, handwriting, walking etc. are more difficult. The above impairments lead to more subtle problems with poor body awareness, that is to say, I find it hard/impossible to be aware of where all the parts of my body are in relation to each other.

- In its most simplistic form, Attention Deficit Disorder, (ADD) as its name suggests, causes inattention and also impulsiveness. I find concentrating a real problem and am completely incapable of concentrating on any one subject for more than a moment, but am not really impulsive. In the case of ADHD (Attention Deficit Hyperactivity Disorder), the person is also hyperactive. If anything, I am underactive rather than overactive (unless I eat peppermint sweets!), but I sometimes have tremendous difficulty in sitting still.

- Autistic Spectrum disorders have a range of 3 central symptoms, which classify someone as suffering from what is more generally referred to as Autism. The 3 symptoms are basically impairments in imagination, social communication and social interaction, plus a strong tendency towards repetitive behaviour. I have impairments of all the above symptoms to various degrees, but how much does the way I perceive 'the world' through my faulty senses affect the way I behave? It seems to me Autistic people have even worse perceptual difficulties over a greater range of senses and systems than Dyslexic, Dyspraxic or ADD sufferers. There are so many combinations of severity under the general title of Autism, that some of these combinations are distinct enough to be given different names; for instance Asperger's Syndrome. After writing this book, in October 1996 I was diagnosed as suffering from Asperger's Syndrome.

I have seen all these main characteristics in each of the above conditions, occurring in varying degrees, in different people. For example, someone may have Dyslexic tendencies whilst another person may suffer very severely from Dyslexia. I also realised that some unfortunate people suffer from more than one of the above to varying degrees and in any combination. For example a person may suffer from Autism and Dyslexia, whilst another person may suffer from Dyslexia and have Dyspraxic tendencies, while yet another may suffer from ADD and have very poor muscle control - Dyspraxic tendencies.

Once I had realised that Dyslexia, Dyspraxia, ADD and Autism were distinct, I also noticed that they seemed paradoxically to be related to each other. There is a huge range of associated symptoms that can occur in any combination in Dyslexia, Dyspraxia, ADD and Autism. Many of these associated symptoms are listed here: allergies & sensitivities, poor articulation, balance problems, concentration & discrimination between stimuli problems, difficulty with comprehending instructions, good and bad days, hearing problems, hypoactive & hyperactive senses, judging distance difficulties, language problems, memory difficulties, poor mental arithmetic, messiness & disorganisation, lack of sense of direction, one-tracked mind, difficulty with orders/sequences, potential phobias, reading difficulties due to defects in vision, language comprehension problems, stress, time disorientation, untidy handwriting, visual and auditory distortions. Additionally, it is reported that some people have been helped by certain medications; does this mean that they have chemical imbalances as well as, or instead of, neurological problems? (I have never tried any such medications.)

Each Dyslexic, Dyspraxic, ADD, Autistic person can have any combination, to varying degrees, of any of the associated symptoms in the above list. Beyond this I realised that many so called 'normal' people very often exhibit to some degree, one or more of the above associated symptoms! Could some of the variations between 'normal' people just be caused by their neurology working in slightly different ways? For instance, some people are unexplainably and continually clumsy, not sporty, poor at fine close work requiring fine muscle control, a bit 'odd', irritated by stripy patterns, read slower than expected or have poor concentration etc, etc...I could carry on for pages!

What else could distorted senses do to a person's ability to cope? It does not take much stretch of the imagination to understand that distorted sensory perceptions of my environment can give a sense of insecurity and fear. For instance, if some of my fears became out of control they could turn me into an agoraphobic[13]. I have come across people, who like myself have the same sort of faulty perception of 'the world'. Their sight, distance perception, hearing, balance, concentration, etc. are distorted, but unlike myself, their compensations broke down and they became agoraphobic before reaching adulthood. It was only the knowledge of my potential to become agoraphobic and then my understanding of my distorted world, which motivated and enabled me to compensate, thus saving me from agoraphobia. I am able to quash my emotional responses and compensate for the distortions, enabling me to understand the reality of a given situation. This means I cope with going outside and to crowded places, without becoming anxious, although I find such environments tiring.

On the next page is an illustration I did while at university. It depicts the view from my window, as I saw it.

---

[13] Agoraphobia is a morbid dread of open spaces (i e anything beyond the front door of a sufferer's house) and is often associated with a fear of crowded places. I am only considering secondary neurosis

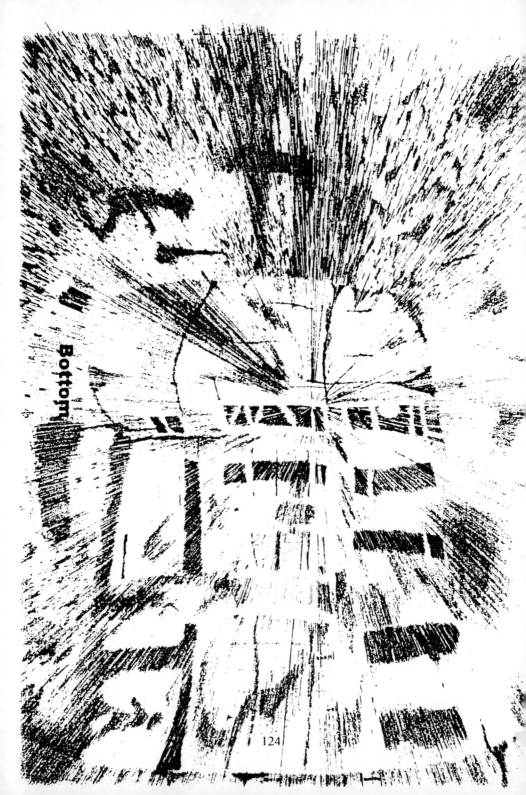

Reflecting on my own experiences I cannot help but wonder: Why Dyslexia, Dyspraxia, ADD and Autism are distinct yet, have a wide range of common characteristics? Why do some people suffer from more than one of these? Why are there so many variations that the exact boundaries between the conditions are not easily definable? Why is there such a range of possible combinations between 'normal' people who have one minor, symptom to severely affected individuals e.g. Autism? Why should so many 'normal' people have one or more of the associated symptoms? Could these associated symptoms result in other medical conditions?

My personal theory of what happens between neurology and psychology of people such as myself, is shown in the diagram on the next page. This is the culmination of my nine years of thinking and is a broad theoretical framework, which is based on my own firsthand experience and observations.

Hale's Syndrome

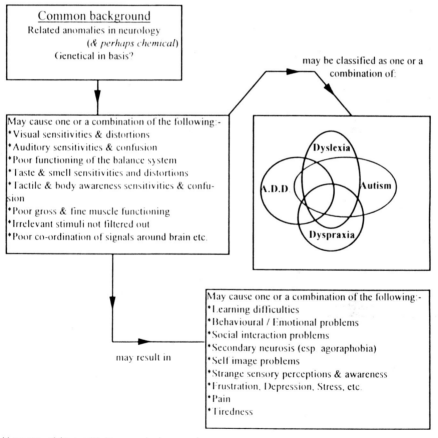

Note: any of the sensitivities may be hyper or hypo

A.D.D. = Attention Deficit Disorder

The combination, number and degree of the defects in the neurological structure will be dependent upon where the dysfunction occurs. The effect of the dysfunction on the person will hinge on their ability to compensate, which is determined by such things as: survival instincts, motivation, determination, courage, intelligence, ingenuity, nurture, stability of childhood, upbringing, high pain threshold, willingness to try and behave/act within the bounds of normality, etc. Often the disability seems to be, at least in part, genetical. I have noticed that many children with these problems have at least one parent (or other family member) with some similar symptoms (not necessarily to the same degree).

I do not have all the answers but simply some insight drawn from my own firsthand experience. I cannot scientifically prove that my diagram is correct, as it has been created from my own casual observations. My gut feelings are no substitute for raw data. My main concern is not whether my diagram is right or wrong, but that the truth is found. Perhaps people like myself have faulty genes that cause us to have subtly different cell structures in our brains, which stop us from developing in the 'normal' way. Do chemical imbalances further complicate the problem? Do messages take the wrong/alternative routes through the brain? Are some parts of the brain under active and other parts over active?

One thing I know without any doubt, is that plenty of further research is needed and I hope this book may encourage someone to take the initiative in this. I would gladly take part in any such research. The result of the research remaining incomplete is that doctors, psychologists, psychiatrists and educationalists are inadvertently causing many children and adults to have either no treatment/help or inappropriate treatment/help, leaving them suffering unnecessarily.

Perhaps undeveloped reflexes are an indicator of a brain with a different structure. Autopsies of people with Dyslexia and Autism show them to have partly different brain cell structures. Do the exercises that are alleged to correct the reflexes, change the cell structure of the brain so that it is 'normal'? Perhaps they could, if all that has happened in people like myself is that we have too many brain cells (because the cells were not shed during the first months of life)? Could there be a part of a gene that is responsible for so many different conditions and symptoms being apparently linked? What part do genes play? Some children are just 'naturally' late learning to read and write and after initial problems continue on to have educationally 'normal' lives. Perhaps these initial problems occur because the required neurological pathways in the brain somehow develop a little late? Why do people like me have minds which apparently think differently? What is thinking? What is consciousness? What is life? If there is a point to our lives, what is it? Do we have the intellectual capacity to understand everything? Why do we exist? Why does 'our' Universe exist?

???????
?????
???
?

2

....September 1995. Academic year spent at home preparing for and writing this book. Preparation for the book involved doing crosswords so that I could learn more about how the English language was manipulated and analysing the construction of television programmes to give me a sense of how a 'story' was constructed. The preparation for writing this book has caused an enormous surge in my ability to find words to express myself. I know that it is the right time to write this book because at last my anger at those who mistreated me, has gone. Knowledge of my problems has made me realise and accept that what has happened was nobody's fault. I have forgiven everybody, including myself. Maybe I can help people in 'the world' to understand the way some of us perceive. Hopefully then, some of the suffering can be alleviated. I am now 26 years old....

I started life confused and unable to make consistent sense of a vast array of things, then grew into a child who was searching for understanding, and onward into a teenager, depressed and distraught over her inability to be 'normal'. As an adult I began to find significant consistency and understanding, and eventually came to realise that I was a part of 'the world'. I have aimed to give an overview of my life, which gives the maximum amount of insight into my different view of the world. I hope my experiences shed enough light on my situation to help others like myself to be better understood by themselves and the people around them. Yes, I have problems. It has taken me 26 years to discover how I perceive, relative to 'normal' people and to teach my immediate family and close friends. For these people, reading this book has been the most powerful account ever given of 'my world' and their new and much deeper understanding of my situation has given me a sense of liberation. At last I am understood.

While I was in my initial years at school, Dyslexia was considered by a great many teachers/professionals to be somehow psychological and/or sociological in nature and was dismissed. Fortunately these days there is much better awareness and more help available. However, I am aware of teachers and other professionals who still wish to take the easy way out, live with their heads buried in the sand and believe that there is not a physical basis to such problems! The outward physical symptoms of Dyslexia are in many cases reasonably easy to identify e.g. poor co-ordination, poor handwriting etc. I consider these to be indications of something different in the way the brain works, rather than a literal inability to learn. It is harder to learn to read if only part of a word is seen at any one time. Likewise it is more difficult to write neatly if the arm and hand do not obey the conscious mind.

In many people such as myself, it is much easier to recognise the psychological and/or educational problems and ignore the possibility of deeper problems such as a different neurological make-up. This does NOT mean all people with psychological abnormalities have a direct physical basis to their problems, it just means beware, because their psychological distress may be the outward result of underlying physical problems.

There was no intuitive way for anyone to know how I perceived, or vice versa. I act in a way that is relative to my senses/environment and this often caused me to behave in ways that deviate from the norm. I had originally assumed that I was the same as everybody else, just as the people I came into contact with assumed I was just unintelligent, slow etc. Without insight or a frame of reference these were natural mistakes. I was the one with the firsthand experience of 'my world' and it was impossible for others looking at me from their usual outside perspective, to understand what I was perceiving on the inside. How could they have understood something that is foreign to them? One thing I am certain of is, there are many different ways of perceiving. This gives me an open-mindedness and a willingness to understand others, who are different from myself, whatever the difference may be.

Discovering the reality of my physical environment was in my case initiated by my experience of differences in the operation of my Central Nervous System, which in turn gave me a frame of reference on which to start my analysis. My search for the truth involved talking to people and very carefully constructing questions to discover what they perceived. Once I had appreciated differences in 'my world' it then became clear that the way I behaved and reacted to my environment was reasonable. Any person who is psychologically 'normal' would have immense problems operating in my hostile physical environment and like myself may feel and/or appear psychologically weak, or in some cases may even develop abnormal behaviour patterns. Is it really that surprising that people like myself are often unable to act in a completely 'normal' fashion? This book could not have been written if I had never deduced where my physical differences lie.

Throughout my life I have had the freedom to investigate my environment. I would not swap that freedom for anything in the world. I can think of nothing worse than my parents being overprotective and wrapping me up in cotton wool. If my parents had done this, I would probably have never done or achieved much, in a sterile environment there would have been little opportunity for me to make any consistent sense of 'my world' and 'the world'. Despite spending most of my life in the extremely difficult situation where nobody has understood me, I would still rather have my life where nobody understands me than lose my freedom and be molly-coddled.

There is not a 'manual' for parents on 'how to make your child turn out right', so my parents just accepted me as being different and providing that I did not act completely inappropriately they gave me freedom to explore. If, when I was a child, my parents had known what they now know, how would they have reacted? I hope that they would have still given me the freedom and made me do a variety of activities, but would have been able to support me when things got tough. Unfortunately, everyone's ignorance often compounded my problems. Through my early teenage years my life was made unbearable by the total lack of understanding my parents had of my predicament, but a little understanding and patience would have gone a long way. Even now I still need support from family and close friends. I do not think they would dare try to molly-coddle me!

This book has been designed to give an insight into a different way of perceiving. I most certainly do not have all the answers and there is no simple solution to overcoming problems such as mine. I have had to work extremely hard at mastering and coming to terms with my difficulties, consequently I would be the first to advocate an easier way, but there is no point in painting an untrue rosy picture. Every person is different and therefore, each must search out the best forms of help and compensations within their own situation. All I can do is give an insight into the ways (and mistakes!) of myself, my family, friends and all those who have come into contact with me.

On a personal level, I am still wondering whether returning to university for the intellectual stimulation, is worth the pain? But, if I do not return to university what shall I do with the rest of my life? Should I do a home study degree course? If I do attain a degree what would I do with it? As an intelligent individual I feel it is my right to be able obtain an honours degree. Perhaps I should forget about studying for a while and instead join the workforce? Maybe I could work from home? Possibly I could obtain an honours degree while holding down a job? Ultimately it is my ambition is to do a Ph.D., work in a research environment and leave my parental home. The answers to these questions are for me to discover and likewise people with similar problems need to find their own personal solutions in life. Hopefully, one day there will be research that will bring about a cure or significant relief, but in the meantime, I believe that all any of us can do is to keep persevering and try to find a sensible way through the labyrinth of life.

Alison

Visit my Web site and try out Sight98 which simulates how I see text on a page

http://www.hale.ndirect.co.uk

please feel free to write to me at Archimedes Press (address on next page)

P.S. *December 1997 - I have now had time to come to terms with the diagnosis of Asperger's Syndrome and am aware of the extent of my problems with understanding* people. Simply knowing that I do not read people, is in itself an enormous asset. I no longer worry about having an idealised normal life; if I get married, have lots of friends, etc. that's fine, if not, I shall not worry. I still believe one of my strongest defences against all my disabilities is the awareness of exactly where my problems lie.

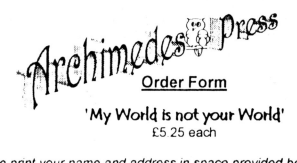

Order Form

'My World is not your World'
£5.25 each

Please print your name and address in space provided below:

First name	
Last name	
Address	
County	
Postal	
Telephone number	

Price (per book) within UK (including P&P) Stg**£5.95**

Pounds Sterling cheques should be made payable to Alison Hale
Special price for three or more copies apply to address below

Please return order form and cheque to:-
        Alison Hale
        Archimedes Press
        Glebe House
        Station Lane
        Ingatestone
        Essex CM4 0BP
        United Kingdom

Tel: 01277 352589